Walking San Francisco

Liz Gans & Rick Newby

A/A Endorsed by the American Volkssport Association

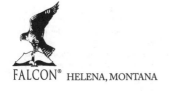

FALCON® HELENA, MONTANA

A FALCON GUIDE®

Falcon® Publishing is continually expanding its list of recreational guidebooks. All books include detailed descriptions, accurate maps, and all the information necessary for enjoyable trips. You can order extra copies of this book and get information and prices for other Falcon® books by writing Falcon, P.O. Box 1718, Helena, MT 59624 or calling toll-free 1-800-582-2665. Also, please ask for a free copy of our current catalog. Visit our website at www.FalconOutdoors.com or contact us by e-mail at falcon@falcon.com.

©1999 by Falcon® Publishing, Inc., Helena, Montana.
Printed in Canada.

Icons of Mexican Art © Hector Escarraman, 1995. All rights reserved.

   3 4 5 6 7 8 9 0 TP 03 02 01 00

Falcon and FalconGuide are registered trademarks of Falcon® Publishing, Inc.

Series editors: Judith Galas and Cindy West.

All black-and-white photos by the authors.

Library of Congress Cataloging-in-Publication Data
Gans, Liz.
    Walking San Francisco / Liz Gans and Rick Newby.
        p.   cm. — (A FalconGuide)
    Includes index.
    ISBN 1-56044-706-0 (pbk.)
    1. Hiking—California—San Francisco Metropolitan Area Guidebooks.
    2. Walking—California—San Francisco Metropolitan Area Guidebooks.
    3. San Francisco Metropolitan Area (Calif.) Guidebooks. I. Newby,
    Rick. II. Title. III. Series: Falcon guide.
    GV199.42.C22S26994 1999
    917.94'610453—dc21   99-28934
                                                                       CIP

CAUTION

Outdoor recreational activities are by their very nature potentially hazardous. All participants in such activities must assume responsibility for their own actions and safety. The information contained in this guidebook cannot replace sound judgment and good decision-making skills, which help reduce exposure, nor does the scope of this book allow for the disclosure of all the potential hazards and risks involved in such activities.

　　Learn as much as possible about the outdoor recreational activities in which you participate, prepare for the unexpected, and be cautious. The reward will be a safer and more enjoyable experience.

 Text pages printed on recycled paper.

For Marg and Joe,
who have walked San Francisco
for more than fifty years

In memoriam

Elaine Isabelle Crowe Newby (1925–1998)

Contents

the walks

Acknowledgments

First, and most of all, we want to thank Margaret and Joe Gans, who encouraged, nurtured, and walked with us while we wrote *Walking San Francisco*. Their home on Telegraph Hill was our San Francisco haven, and their enthusiasm for this project was boundless.

We want to thank the wonderful Bay Area friends and acquaintances who took us into their homes, gave us hot tips for good restaurants, intriguing attractions, and great walks—and sometimes tested the walks for us: Richard Gans; Peter Merts; Michele Foyer and Mark Fredenburg; Peter Rutledge Koch; Harold Charns and Rose Schubert; John Palmer and Leslie Cobb; Gilda and Gregory Loew; Linda Maki and Doug, Nathan, and Aaron Groom; Bob Hoover; Anne Appleby and Melissa Kwasny; Ed Gilbert; Griff and Chris Williams; Gary and Karen Carson; Paul and Sandra Tsang; and John and Trish Kinsella.

We owe a special debt of gratitude to Jennifer Thompson, who helped us see San Francisco with sharper eyes. Thanks, too, to J. M. Cooper and Peter Merts for invaluable photographic advice, and to Adolph Gasser, Inc., Third Eye Photographics, and Jeff Van Tine for their darkroom magic.

Julie Soller, public relations coordinator at the San Francisco Convention and Visitors Bureau, gave us helpful guidance, as did Kathleen Mozena, of the bureau's membership office. Paul McBride of Wheelchairs of Berkeley graciously helped us decide which of our walks are truly wheelchair accessible. Anita Hill, executive director of Yerba Buena Alliance, kept us up-to-date on developments in the Yerba Buena Gardens. Bob Yeargin of City Guides pointed out many of the sights we mention in our Chinatown walk; and Patricia Rose, Precita Eyes Mural Arts Center, showed us the Mission's rich mural heritage. In Ina Coolbrith Park, Charles the Thinker offered spiritual advice and several walk ideas. And Jeanne Fidler told us much about the bird life of the Marin Headlands.

We want also to offer our gratitude to the many folks at the Golden Gate National Recreation Area (GGNRA) who unstintingly provided guidance about particular walks in the GGNRA. These include Dean J. Whittaker, Presidio Visitor Center; Bob G. Holloway, Cliff House Visitor Center; J. Sherman, Baker Beach; and Cathy Petrick and Diana Roberts, Marin Headlands Visitor Center. Carol Prince, Golden Gate National Parks Association, graciously guided us through the changes underway along the Golden Gate Promenade. And special thanks to Chris Powell of the Golden Gate National Recreation Area, who oversaw the review of all walks within the GGNRA, and to John Cunnane, supervisory park ranger at the San Francisco Maritime National Historical Park, who reviewed our Fisherman's Wharf walk.

Our editor, Judith Galas, was a consummate professional throughout, and her clear and savvy direction made the research and writing of *Walking San Francisco* a real joy. Gayle Shirley, our enthusiastic editor at Falcon Publishing, provided great advice and was infinitely patient. Our thanks to two wonderful editors.

Finally, our gratitude to Randall Green, former Falcon guidebook editor, who signed us up for this project, and to Bill Schneider and Chris Cauble, who made it happen.

Foreword

For more than twenty years, Falcon has guided millions of people to America's wild outside, showing them where to paddle, hike, bike, bird, fish, climb, and drive. With this walking series, we at Falcon ask you to try something just as adventurous. We invite you to experience this country from its sidewalks, not its back roads, and to stroll through some of America's most interesting cities.

In their haste to get where they are going, travelers often bypass this country's cities, and in the process, they miss the historic and scenic treasures hidden among the bricks. Many people seek spectacular scenery and beautiful settings on top of the mountains, along the rivers, and in the woods. While nothing can replace the serenity and inspiration of America's natural wonders, we should not overlook the beauty of the urban landscape.

The steel and glass of municipal mountains reflect the sunlight and make people feel small in the shadows. Birds sing in city parks, water burbles in the fountains, and along the sidewalks walkers can still see abundant wildlife—their fellow human beings.

Falcon's many outdoor guidebooks have encouraged people not only to explore and enjoy America's natural beauty but to preserve and protect it. Our cities also are meant to be enjoyed and explored, and their irreplaceable treasures need care and protection.

When travelers and walkers want to explore something that is inspirational and beautiful, we hope they will lace up their walking shoes and point their feet toward one of this country's many cities.

For there, along the walkways, they are sure to discover the excitement, history, beauty, and charm of urban America.

—*The Editors*

Preface: Come Walk San Francisco

San Francisco is one of this earth's mythical cities, fabled for its gorgeous natural setting, its urbanity, and the charm of its distinctive neighborhoods. Mild in climate and quirky in character, the city greets each visitor with an abundance of attractions and opportunities.

For the walker, it offers challenging topography—all those hills!—and breathtaking vistas. It is a compact city, and an ambitious pedestrian can see much in a single day, traversing a startling array of cultures and microclimates. For the hungry walker, this culinary city boasts more than 3,000 restaurants, many of them world-class.

And besides its own network of city parks—including that wonderland, Golden Gate Park—San Francisco is home to the Golden Gate National Recreation Area (GGNRA). The largest urban national park in the world, the GGNRA stretches beyond San Francisco, to Alcatraz Island and Muir Woods, while including some of the city's most beloved places, from the Cliff House to the Presidio.

Walking San Francisco takes full advantage of the GGNRA, featuring eight walks within the park's boundaries. These walks, mostly in natural areas, stand in striking contrast to those inside the city itself. Imagine: One day you are walking along vibrant, crowded Fisherman's Wharf, and the next, you find quiet on a forest trail in the Presidio. Another day you explore the rich cultures of Chinatown or the Mission District, and the next you are striding along the Coastal Trail on Lands End. And then, for a change of pace, you spend a morning wandering history-rich Fort Point and the afternoon stalking the slopes of Pacific Heights, in search of the city's most photogenic Victorian architecture.

San Francisco has been called the loveliest city on earth. Discover this truth for yourself. Try *Walking San Francisco*.

Map Legend

Walk Route (paved)		Interstate	(80)
Walk Route (unpaved)		U.S. Highway	{101}
Streets and Roads		State and County Roads	(1)
Tunnel		Start/Finish of Loop Walk	S/F
Hiking/Walking Trail		Parking Area	P
Building		Ocean or Lake	
Church or Cathedral		Park/Open Space	
Restrooms, Male and Female		Bridge	
Handicapped Access		Cable Car	
Beach		Cable Car Turnaround	
Picnic Area		Park Gate	
Playground		Elevation	✕ Hill 88
Tennis Courts		Map Orientation	N
Baseball Field		Scale of Distance	0 0.5 1 Miles
Stairs			

San Franciso Map Overview

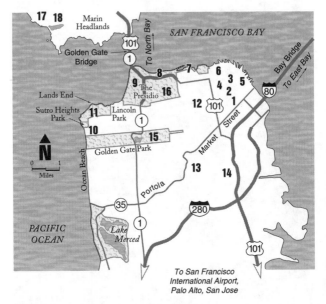

Boldface numbers are walk locations.

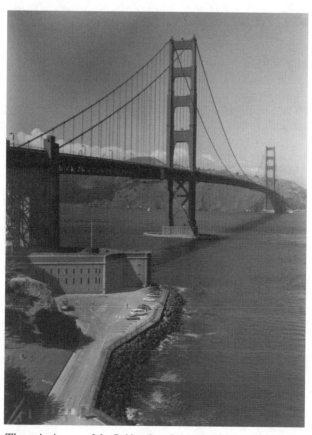

The majestic span of the Golden Gate Bridge, with historic Fort Point nestled beneath its south end, links San Francisco to Marin County and points north.

Introduction

Walking the streets and boulevards of a city can take you into its heart and give you a feel for its pulse and personality. From the sidewalk looking up, you can appreciate its architecture. From the sidewalk peeking in, you can find the quaint shops, local museums, and great eateries that give a city its charm and personality. From its nature paths, you can smell the flowers, glimpse the wildlife, gaze at a lake, or hear a creek gurgle. Only by walking can you get close enough to read the historical plaques and watch the people. When you walk a city, you get it all—adventure, scenery, local color, good exercise, and fun.

How to use this guide

We have designed this book so that you can easily find the walks that match your interests, time, and energy level. The Trip Planner (see pages 8 and 9) is the first place you should look when deciding on a walk. This table will give you the basic information—a walk's distance, the estimated walking time, and the difficulty. The pictures or icons in the table also tell you specific things about the walk:

Every walk has something of interest, but this icon tells you that the route will have particular appeal to the shutterbug. So bring your camera. You will have great views of the city or the surrounding area, and you are likely to get some wonderful scenic shots.

Somewhere along the route you will have the chance to get food or a beverage. You will have to glance through the walk description to determine where and what kind of food and beverages are available. Walks that do not have the food icon probably are along nature trails or in noncommercial areas of the city.

1

During your walk you will have the chance to shop. More detailed descriptions of the types of stores you will find can be found in the actual walk description.

This walk features something kids will enjoy seeing or doing—a park, zoo, museum, or play equipment. In most cases the walks that carry this icon are short and follow an easy, fairly level path. You know your young walking companions best. If your children are patient walkers who do not tire easily, then feel free to choose walks that are longer and harder. In fact, depending on a child's age and energy, most children can do any of the walks in this book. The icon only notes those walks we think they will especially enjoy.

Your path will take you primarily through urban areas. Buildings, small city parks, and paved paths are what you will see and pass.

You will pass through a large park or walk in a natural setting where you can see and enjoy nature.

The wheelchair icon means that the path is fully accessible. This walk would be easy for someone pushing a wheelchair or stroller. We have made every attempt to follow a high standard for accessibility. The icon means there are curb cuts or ramps along the entire route, plus a wheelchair-accessible bathroom somewhere along the way. The path is mostly or entirely paved, and ramps and unpaved surfaces are clearly described. If you use a wheelchair and have the ability to negotiate curbs and dirt paths or to wheel for longer distances and on uneven surfaces, you may want to skim the directions for the walks that do not carry this symbol. You may find other walks you will enjoy. If in doubt, read the full text of the walk or call the contact source for guidance.

At the start of each walk description, you will find specific information describing the route and what you can expect on your walk:

General location: Here you will get the walk's general location in the city or within a specific area.

Special attractions: Look here to find the specific things you will pass. If this walk has museums, historic homes, restaurants, or wildlife, it will be noted here.

Difficulty rating: We have designed or selected walking routes that an ordinary person in reasonable health can complete. The walks are rated from 1 to 5, 1 being the easiest. But the ease or difficulty does not relate to a person's level of physical fitness. A walk with a rating of 5 can be completed by an average walker, but that walker may feel tired when he or she has completed the walk and may feel some muscle soreness.

How easy or hard a walk may be depends on each person. But here are some general guidelines of what the number rating indicates:

A walk rated as Easy/1 is flat, with few or no hills. Most likely you will be walking on a maintained surface made of concrete, asphalt, wood, or packed earth. The path will be easy to follow, and you will be only a block or so from a phone, other people, or businesses. If the walk is less than a mile, you may be able to walk comfortably in street shoes.

A walk rated as Moderate/3 includes some hills, and a few may be quite steep. Portions of the path may include stretches of sand, dirt, gravel, or small crushed rock; the single walk with this rating in *Walking San Francisco* is mostly on pavement, but involves a good deal of climbing. You should wear walking shoes.

A walk rated as Difficult/5 probably has an unpaved path

that includes rocks, tree roots, and patches of vegetation. The trail may have steep ups and downs, and you may have to pause now and then to interpret the walk directions against the natural setting. Carrying water is advisable, and you may be alone for long stretches of the walk. Walking shoes are a must, and hiking boots may be helpful.

Walks rated 2 and 4 fall somewhere in between. For example, three walks in this guide are rated Moderate/2, meaning that—while they are at least partially on nonpaved surfaces and include some hills—they are not as challenging as the single walk rated Moderate/3. We have rated three walks in this guide as Difficult/4, even though they are entirely on pavement, because they involve climbing extremely steep streets and stairways. If you are in doubt, read the walk text carefully or call the listed contact for more information.

Distance and estimated time: This gives the total distance of the walk. The time allotted for each walk is based on walking time only, which we have calculated at about 30 minutes per mile, a slow pace. Most people have no trouble walking a mile in half an hour, and people with some walking experience often walk a 20-minute mile. If the walk includes museums, shops, or restaurants, you may want to add sightseeing time to the estimate.

Services: Here you will find out if such things as restrooms, parking, refreshments, or information centers are available and where you are likely to find them.

Restrictions: The most often noted restriction is pets, which almost always have to be leashed in a city. Most cities also have strict "pooper-scooper" laws, and they enforce them. But restrictions may also include the hours or days a museum or business is open, age requirements, or whether you can ride a bike on the path. If there is something you cannot do on this walk, it will be noted here.

For more information: Each walk includes at least one contact source for you to call for more information. If an agency or business is named as a contact, you will find its phone number and address in Appendix B. This appendix also includes contact information for any business or agency mentioned anywhere in the book.

Getting started: Here you will find specific directions to the starting point. Most walks are closed loops, which means they begin and end at the same point. Thus, you do not have to worry about finding your car or your way back to the bus stop when your walk is over.

In those cities with excellent transportation, such as San Francisco, it may be easy—and sometimes even more interesting—to end a few of your walks away from the starting point. When this happens, you will get clear directions on how to take public transportation back to your starting point.

If a walk is not a closed loop, this section will tell you where the walk ends, and you will find the exact directions back to your starting point at the end of the walk's directions.

Some downtown walks can be started at any one of several hotels the walk passes. The directions will be for the main starting point, but this section will tell you if it is possible to pick up the walk at other locations. If you are staying at a downtown hotel, it is likely that a walk passes in front of or near your hotel's entrance.

Public transportation: Many cities have excellent transportation systems; others have limited services. If it is possible to take a bus or commuter train to the walk's starting point, you will find the bus or train noted here. You may also find some information about where the bus or train stops.

Overview: Every part of a city has a story. Here is where you will find the story or stories about the people, neighborhoods, and history connected to your walk.

The walk

When you reach this point, you are ready to start walking. In this section you will find not only specific and detailed directions, but you will also learn more about the things you are passing. Those who want only the directions and none of the extras can find the straightforward directions by looking for the ➤.

What to wear

The best advice is to wear something comfortable. Leave behind anything that binds, pinches, rides up, falls down, slips off the shoulder, or comes undone. Otherwise, let common sense, the weather, and your own body tell you what to wear.

What to take

Be sure to take water. Strap a bottle to your fanny pack or tuck a small one in a pocket. If you are walking several miles with a dog, remember to take a small bowl so your pet can have a drink, too.

Carry some water even if you will be walking where refreshments are available. Several small sips taken throughout a walk are more effective than one large drink at the walk's end. Avoid drinks with caffeine or alcohol because they deplete rather than replenish your body's fluids.

Safety and street savvy

Mention a big city and many people immediately think of safety. Is it safe to walk there during the day? What about at night? Are there areas I should avoid?

You should use common sense whether you are walking in a small town or a big city, but safety does not have to be your overriding concern. American cities are enjoyable places, and you will find that they are generally safe places.

Any safety mishap in a large city is likely to involve petty theft or vandalism. So, the biggest tip is simple: Do not tempt thieves. Purses dangling on shoulder straps or slung over your arm, wallets peeking out of pockets, arms burdened with packages, valuables on the car seat—all of these things attract the pickpocket, purse snatcher, or thief. If you look like you could easily be relieved of your possessions, you may be.

Do not carry a purse. Put your money in a money belt or tuck your wallet into a deep side pocket of your pants or skirt or in a fanny pack that rides over your hip or stomach. Lock your valuables in the trunk of your car before you park and leave for your walk. Protect your camera by wearing the strap across your chest, not just over your shoulder. Better yet, put your camera in a backpack.

You also will feel safer if you remember the following:

• Be aware of your surroundings and the people near you.

• Avoid parks or other isolated places at night.

• Walk with others.

• Walk in well-lit and well-traveled areas.

The walks in this book were selected by people who had safety in mind. No walk will take you through a bad neighborhood or into an area of the city that is known to be dangerous. So relax and enjoy your walk.

Trip Planner

Walk name	Difficulty	Distance (miles)	Time	♿	🏙	🌳	👥	📦	☕	📷
Heart of the City										
1. Downtown	easy/1	2.5	1.25 hrs		✓		✓	✓	✓	
2. Chinatown	easy/1	1.5	1 hr		✓		✓	✓	✓	✓
3. North Beach	difficult/4	2	1.5 hrs		✓			✓	✓	✓
4. Russian Hill	difficult/4	3	2.25 hrs		✓			✓	✓	✓
Along the Bay										
5. The Embarcadero	easy/1	3	1.5 hrs	✓	✓		✓	✓	✓	✓
6. Fisherman's Wharf	easy/1	2.5	1.25 hrs	✓	✓		✓	✓	✓	✓
7. Marina Green	easy/1	3–3.8	1.5–2 hrs	✓	✓	✓	✓	✓	✓	✓
8. Golden Gate Promenade	easy/1	3.5	2 hrs	✓		✓	✓			✓
Pacific Coast										
9. Golden Gate Bridge and Baker Beach	moderate/2	3	1.5 hrs			✓	✓		✓	✓
10. Ocean Beach	easy/1	1.25	45 min	✓		✓	✓		✓	✓
11. Lands End	moderate/2	3	1.5 hrs			✓	✓			✓

Other Distinctive Neighborhoods

				Wheelchair access	City setting	Nature setting	Good for kids	Shopping	Food	Bring camera
12. Pacific Heights and Japantown	moderate/3	2.5	1.25 hrs		✓			✓	✓	✓
13. The Castro District and Noe Valley	difficult/4	4	2 hrs		✓			✓	✓	✓
14. Mission Murals	easy/1	2	1 hr		✓		✓			✓

Parklands

				Wheelchair access	City setting	Nature setting	Good for kids	Shopping	Food	Bring camera
15. Golden Gate Park	easy/1	3.75	2 hrs	✓		✓	✓		✓	✓
16. The Presidio	moderate/2	2	1 hr	✓		✓	✓			✓
17. Marin Headlands: Wolf Ridge Loop	difficult/5	5.5	3 hrs			✓				✓
18. Marin Headlands: Rodeo Lagoon	easy/1	1.25	45 min	✓		✓	✓		✓	✓

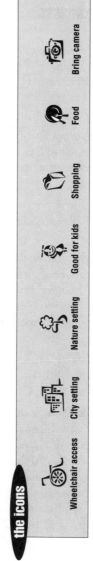

the icons

Wheelchair access   City setting   Nature setting   Good for kids   Shopping   Food   Bring camera

Meet San Francisco

General
County: San Francisco
Time Zone: Pacific
Area Code: 415

Size
Nation's fifth largest metropolitan region
758,987 people within city limits
6.5 million in metro area
11.4 million visitors annually
46 square miles

Elevation
Sea level to 938 feet above sea level

Climate
Average yearly precipitation: 19.33 inches
Average relative humidity, early morning: 85.8 percent
Average relative humidity, midday: 64 percent
Maximum average temperature: 62.5 degrees F
Minimum average temperature: 51 degrees F

Major highways
Interstates: I-80; I-280
U.S. highways: US 101
State highways: CA 1; CA 35

Airport service (San Francisco and Oakland)
Aces Airline, Aer Lingus, Aeroflot, Aerolineas Argentinas, Air Afrique, Air Canada, Air France, Air Malta, Air New Zealand, Alaska, Aloha, America West, American, American Trans Air, Asiana, Avianca, Aviateca, British Airlines, Bwia International, Canadian Airlines, Cathay Pacific, Cayman Airways, China Airlines, City Bird, Continental, Delta, Egypt Air, El Al Israel Airlines, Emirates, Finnair,

Frontier, Garuda Indonesia, Hawaiian, Horizon, Iberia, Japan Airlines, KLM Royal Dutch, Korean Air, LTU International, Lufthansa, Malaysia Airlines, Martinair Holland, Mexicana, Midwest Express, Northwest, Pakistan International, Pan American, Philippine Airlines, Qantas, Reno Air, Sabena Belgian, Shanghai Airlines, Shuttle by United, Singapore Airlines, Southwest, Swissair, Taca International, Thai Airways, TWA, United, Vanguard, Varig Brazilian, Virgin Atlantic, Western Pacific, Yemen Airlines

Rail service
Amtrak
Caltrain
Bay Area Rapid Transit (BART)

Bus service
Alameda-Contra Costa Transit District (AC Transit)
Golden Gate Transit
Green Tortoise Sleeper Coaches
Greyhound
SamTrans
San Francisco Municipal Railway (Muni)

Ferry service
Blue & Gold Fleet, Golden Gate Ferry

Major industries
Tourism, recreation, retailing, transportation, publishing, technology, finance, construction, and food.

Recreation
San Francisco is park-rich, with more than 1,000 city, county, and state parks, recreation centers, swimming pools, public works of art, and stairways, plus the Golden Gate National Recreation Area, the largest urban national park in the world at 76,500 acres and 28 miles of coastline.

Media

Television stations

KBHK (UPN)—Channel 44
KCNS (Independent; Chinese language)—Channel 38
KDTV (UNI; Spanish language)—Channel 14
KGO (ABC)—Channel 7
KPIX (CBS)—Channel 5
KMTP (Independent)—Channel 32
KPST (Independent; Chinese language)—Channel 66
KRON (NBC)—Channel 4
KTSF (Independent)—Channel 26
KTVU (Fox)—Channel 2
KQED (PBS)—Channel 9
KBWB (WBN)—Channel 20

Radio stations

Many stations, including:

KABL 960 AM—Pop standards
KKHI 1510 AM—Classical
KCBS 740 AM—All news
KGO 810 AM—News, talk, and sports
KVTO 1400 AM—Asian
KIQI 1010 AM—Spanish
KSOL 98.9 FM—Spanish
KUSF 90.3 FM—Alternative music
KCSM 91.1 FM—Jazz
KQED 88.5 FM—National Public Radio
KPOO 89.5 FM—Listener-sponsored
KALW 91.7 FM—National Public Radio, BBC, CBC

Newspapers

The Independent, San Francisco Bay Guardian, San Francisco Chronicle, San Francisco Examiner, SF Weekly, and more than 50 others, including papers in Chinese, Japanese, Korean, Spanish, German, and Russian.

Special annual events

- January: Berlin and Beyond Film Festival, Dr. Martin Luther King, Jr., Birthday Celebration, Festival of Lights at Fisherman's Wharf.

- February: California International Antiquarian Book Fair, Chinese New Year Parade and Celebration, San Francisco Arts of Pacific Asia Show, San Francisco Tribal, Folk & Textile Art Show.

- March: San Francisco Flower and Garden Show, San Francisco International Asian American Film Festival, Whole Life Expo.

- April: Cherry Blossom Festival, San Francisco International Film Festival.

- May: Carnaval in the Mission, Cinco de Mayo, San Francisco Youth Arts Festival.

- June: Ethnic Dance Festival, Haight Street Fair, Juneteenth Celebration, North Beach Festival, Old Harbor Festival, San Francisco Gay/Lesbian/Transgender Pride Celebration Parade, Street Performers Festival, Union Street Spring Festival Arts & Crafts Fair.

- July: Books by the Bay, Folk Art to Funk, Jazz & All That Art on Fillmore, Jewish Film Festival, San Francisco Chronicle Fourth of July Waterfront Festival, Stern Grove Midsummer Music Festival.

- August: American Craft Council Craft Fair, African-Solo Performance Festival, Comedy Celebration Day, Nihonmachi Street Fair, Renaissance Pleasure Faire.

- September: Absolut a la Carte, A la Park, Autumn Moon Festival, Blues & Art Festival, Festival de las Americas, Festival of the Sea, Folsom Street Fair, San

13

Francisco Blues Festival, San Francisco Fringe Festival, San Francisco International Art Exposition, San Francisco Shakespeare Festival.

- October: Exotic Erotic Ball, Halloween San Francisco, International Vintage Poster Fair, Italian Heritage Parade and Festival, San Francisco Antiques Show, San Francisco Jazz Festival.

- November: American Indian Film Festival, Cafe Arts Month, Film Arts Festival of Independent Cinema, Grand National Rodeo, Horse and Stock Show, Harvest Festival and Christmas Crafts Show, San Francisco Bay Area Book Festival, San Francisco International Automobile Show, The Great San Francisco Snow Party.

- December: Festival of Lights at Fisherman's Wharf, Christmas at Sea.

Weather

San Francisco's nearly always temperate climate makes the city ideal for walking. With temperatures seldom dipping below 40 degrees F and rarely rising above 70—though there is an occasional hot day—walking San Francisco is almost always cool and pleasant. Of course, you may think differently if your legs are not quite up to the legendary hills or if you get caught in a heavy rainstorm without an umbrella. Hint: When in doubt, carry a small umbrella in your jacket pocket, rucksack, or briefcase.

Weather-wise, spring and fall are the best times to visit the city by the bay. December, January, and February are often rainy, and summer days, oddly enough, can chill you to the bone with their wind and fog. Of course, most visitors come to San Francisco in the summer anyway, another reason to visit in glorious October or radiant May—when the usual tourist spots are less crowded.

Because of its many hills, this city has several distinct microclimates. From the often foggy Ocean Beach to the sunny Mission District, San Francisco weather can shift moods within a few blocks. This means being prepared for a range of eventualities. Always carry that umbrella, and wear several layers—San Francisco is the quintessential sweater city.

Transportation

By car: San Francisco is a challenging place to drive a car—steep hills, often narrow streets, tremendous competition for on-street parking, and rush-hour traffic compounded by bridge-crossing bottlenecks to the north and east of the city. We heartily recommend stowing your car and relying on public transportation. Traffic is heaviest from 7 to 10 A.M. and 4 to 7 P.M., but it seems to be getting thicker and thicker at all hours of the day.

There are four major freeway approaches into San Francisco:

U.S. Highway 101 South leads from the **North Bay** across the **Golden Gate Bridge** and then through San Francisco on three city streets—Lombard Street, Van Ness Avenue, and South Van Ness Avenue. It resumes as a freeway several blocks south of Market Street and continues on southward, past the San Francisco International Airport to the San Francisco Peninsula.

Conversely, **U.S. Highway 101 North** is a major highway into San Francisco from the **San Francisco Peninsula** to the south. From US 101 North you can exit onto Interstate 80 East to travel through San Francisco—above the South of Market area—toward the Bay Bridge.

Interstate 80 West runs from the **East Bay** across the **Bay Bridge** and travels through the city above the South of Market area. It then flows into US 101 North, which heads up Van Ness Avenue toward the Golden Gate Bridge, and into US 101 South, which runs down the San Francisco Peninsula.

Interstate 280 North heads north from the **San Francisco Peninsula** directly into San Francisco's South of Market area. I-280 North is often less congested than US 101 North, and its main exit into downtown San Francisco is easier to negotiate.

The following list of exits may assist you in driving to the start of the walks:

U.S. Highway 101 South:

- 25th Avenue—for going into the Presidio or for reaching Ocean Beach via the east-west artery of Geary Street

- 19th Avenue/Park Presidio—for traveling on California Highway 1 through San Francisco via Park Presidio Boulevard and 19th Avenue and then south to the San Francisco Peninsula

- Marina—for reaching the Marina Green and Fisherman's Wharf

- Downtown/Lombard—for continuing on US 101 South through San Francisco via Lombard Street and Van Ness Avenue

Interstate 80 West:

- Harrison Street/Embarcadero, the first left exit after crossing the Bay Bridge—for going to the Embarcadero to reach the Ferry Building and Fisherman's Wharf

- Fremont Street, the first right exit after crossing the Bay Bridge—for reaching the intersection of Market, Fremont, and Front Streets near the Embarcadero Center and the Ferry Building, and for reaching the intersection of Market, Third, Kearny, and Geary Streets near Union Square

- Fifth Street, the second left exit after crossing the Bay Bridge—for going to the intersection of Market, Third, Kearny, and Geary Streets near Union Square, or to the Fifth & Mission/Yerba Buena Gardens Garage on Fifth

- Ninth Street/Civic Center—for reaching the intersection of Market, Ninth, Hayes, and Larkin Streets near the Civic Center

- US 101 North/Golden Gate Bridge—for reaching Golden Gate Park via US 101 North's Fell/Laguna exit, and for going to the Golden Gate Bridge via US 101 North on Van Ness Avenue

U.S. Highway 101 North:

- I-280 North—for reaching the intersection of Market, Third, Kearny, and Geary Streets near Union Square via I-280 North's Sixth Street exit

- Ninth Street/Civic Center—for reaching the intersection of Market, Ninth, Hayes, and Larkin Streets near the Civic Center

- Fell/Laguna—for going to Golden Gate Park on Fell Street

- I-80 East/Bay Bridge—for reaching the intersection of Market, Third, Kearny, and Geary Streets near Union Square via I-80 East's Fourth Street exit, which is the last exit before you cross the Bay Bridge

Interstate 280 North:

- Golden Gate Bridge/19th Avenue—for reaching Golden Gate Park, the east-west artery of Geary Street, and the Golden Gate Bridge

- US 101 North—for reaching the intersection of Market, Ninth, Larkin, and Hayes via US 101 North's

Ninth Street/Civic Center exit, and for going to Golden Gate Park via US 101 North's Fell/Laguna exit

• Sixth Street—for reaching the intersection of Market, Third, Kearny, and Geary Streets near Union Square, and for going along Bryant Street to the Embarcadero and Fisherman's Wharf. It is also quite simple to get from Sixth Street to the intersection of Market, Ninth, Hayes, and Larkin Streets near the Civic Center.

By bus: San Francisco has an excellent mass transit system known as the San Francisco Municipal Railway (Muni). The city's residents love to complain about Muni's relatively minor glitches; but it is quite reliable, one of the best in the United States. The system includes a fleet of electric- and diesel-powered buses that covers the entire city; the underground Muni Metro, a light-rail system which does not run as smoothly as it might; and the cable cars and streetcars discussed below.

When you first arrive in San Francisco, pick up a current Muni schedule and map, both available from the San Francisco Convention and Visitors Bureau at Hallidie Plaza or selected merchants. With these in hand, you will find traversing the city by bus, light-rail, or streetcar a cinch. In fact, because of the city's shortage of parking, we recommend using public transportation to reach most of our walks. Many bus lines have wheelchair lifts. Call Muni for more details about accessibility.

Several regional bus lines link San Francisco with surrounding communities. Alameda-Contra Costa Transit District (AC Transit) buses run between San Francisco's Transbay Terminal and Western Alameda and Contra Costa Counties in the East Bay. Golden Gate Transit buses cover Marin, Sonoma, San Francisco, and Contra Costa Counties. SamTrans serves San Mateo County with connections to Hayward, Palo Alto, and San Francisco's Transbay Terminal.

Greyhound, and that holdover from hippie days, Green Tortoise Sleeper Coaches, are the commercial long-distance bus lines that serve the city.

By cable car or streetcar: San Francisco's cable cars are among its most famous features, and any visit to the city is incomplete without a ride on one of these colorful anachronisms. Still a functioning part of the San Francisco Municipal Railway (Muni), the cable cars run on three separate lines: the Powell-Hyde, Powell-Mason, and California Street lines. Contact Muni for ticket prices and schedules. And for more information about the history of the city's cable car system, visit the Cable Car Barn and Museum at 1201 Mason Street, on the edge of Chinatown; see Appendix A for more details.

San Francisco also maintains several streetcar lines, powered by an overhead electric cable. Contact Muni for information.

By air: Always expanding, San Francisco International Airport is one of the world's great airfields, at last count the seventh busiest on earth. Airlines from all over the world land here. Scattered throughout the vast airport, intriguing exhibits—ranging from displays of African folk art to a history of the platform shoe—reflect the many cultures that meet here.

We have found that shuttles—there are several companies—provide reliable, relatively inexpensive service to San Francisco. Buses are less expensive than the shuttles but do not take you to your door, and taxis cost nearly twice as much.

Metropolitan Oakland International Airport, across the Bay Bridge, is smaller and just as close to downtown San Francisco as the city's own airport, about 25 minutes when traffic is not too heavy. Again, shuttles are a safe bet, although there is a designated bus—known as AirBART—that will take you to the nearest BART station for a quick underground jaunt into the city.

By train: Amtrak does not cross the bay to San Francisco, but you can find Amtrak passenger stations in nearby Oakland, in Jack London Square at 245 Second Street; in Emeryville, at 5885 Landregan Street; and in Richmond, in the Richmond BART station at McDonald and 16th Streets. Amtrak buses bring passengers from these stations to and from San Francisco. Call Amtrak for details.

Bay Area Rapid Transit (BART) trains serve much of San Francisco, carrying commuters to and from East Bay cities like Oakland and Berkeley—and providing a fast, alternate way to travel from downtown to the Mission District.

Caltrain provides commuter rail service between San Francisco and communities to the south as far as Gilroy, with bus service continuing to Santa Cruz.

By ferry: Although the Golden Gate and Bay Bridges have replaced ferries for most commuters, some San Francisco workers—and tourists—still take ferries across San Francisco Bay. Departing from Pier 41, ferries will take you to Alameda/Oakland, Alcatraz, Angel Island, Sausalito, Tiburon, and Vallejo. Other ferries depart from the Ferry Building or nearby Pier 1, going to Sausalito, Tiburon, Vallejo, Alameda, Oakland, and Larkspur.

Safety

San Francisco is a friendly city, despite its size, and San Franciscans take great delight in sharing their love for—and intimate knowledge of—their city with visitors. At the same time, San Francisco is a big city, with the crime that comes with any large metropolitan area.

Let your common sense be your guide as you walk, and if you have concerns about a particular neighborhood or route, check with friends who live here or ask at the San Francisco Convention and Visitors Bureau. We selected the walks in this book because they offer enjoyable walking experiences in lively and interesting areas that are also safe. If you depart a walk route, be aware that the character of a neighborhood can change within a few blocks.

In general, it is best to walk during daylight so you can read your map and guidebook, enjoy the sights, and watch for uneven surfaces on the sidewalk or trail. We particularly recommend that you not take any of our Parklands or Pacific Coast walks after dark. In fact, all of our walks, we feel, are best undertaken during the daylight hours. And on the less populated walks—Parklands and Pacific Coast walks—we recommend that you always go with a partner.

If you do find yourself walking after dark, be sure to avoid alleyways, parks, and parking lots. When possible, walk with other people and choose well-lit thoroughfares.

A special note for water lovers: Swim only at beaches or pools with lifeguards. The ocean swells can catch you off guard and be extremely dangerous.

For a general review of city safety information, read the tips on page 6. Enjoy your walks in this wonderful city.

The Story of San Francisco

San Francisco, perhaps more than most cities, has benefited from a magnificent natural setting. With its great natural harbor, its temperate climate, and its proximity to prime agricultural lands and rich mineral deposits, it has—from its very beginnings—been a city destined for wealth, power, and beauty.

Ironically, the first humans to walk here—the Coast Miwok and Ohlone Indian tribes—considered the site of present-day San Francisco inhospitable. Faced with the site's seemingly endless sand dunes, windswept cliffs, and impossibly steep hills, these hunter-gatherers found life more pleasant elsewhere in the Bay Area, where they thrived on plentiful game, fish, and edible wild plants.

And European seafarers had their own problems with the place: From the first Spanish sailor to explore the California coast in 1542 to the Spanish, English, and Russian captains who sailed along this rugged shore for the next 200 years, they could not find the entrance—later dubbed the Golden Gate—to San Francisco Bay.

It was not until 1769 that Spaniard Gaspar de Portola stumbled upon the great bay while traveling overland. And finally in 1775, Juan Manuel de Ayala, commanding the *San Carlos,* became the first European to sail through the Golden Gate. Ayala's men thoroughly explored and mapped the bay, realizing that they had discovered a well-sheltered harbor of world-class proportions.

The first Spanish settlers arrived in 1776. In that year, they established a military presence—a presidio—on the windy site of present-day Fort Point. They founded a Franciscan mission—today known as Mission Dolores—three miles to the southeast, in a valley sheltered from the wind and with plenty of water. First named "Yerba Buena" or "good herb" after a creeping mint known for its healing properties, San Francisco marked its founding with a Catholic mass on June 29, 1776, only five days before the ratification of the Declaration of Independence.

As old and as young as the American republic, San Francisco grew slowly at first. Not long a Spanish outpost, it became a part of Mexico following Mexican independence in 1821. And on July 9, 1846, soon after war had broken out between Mexico and the United States, a small American force took possession of Yerba Buena. San Francisco was suddenly American property—just in time for a gold rush that would transform the tiny community by the bay.

With the discovery of gold throughout much of California, San Francisco became a rough-and-ready boomtown overnight. Its grand harbor filled with ships abandoned as their crews headed for the hills, struck by gold fever. The town's population shot from 500 hardy souls in 1846 to 20,000 by the end of 1849. In an economy where gold was plentiful and merchandise of any sort in limited supply, the city's entrepreneurs made instant fortunes. Its population was made up mostly of single men, and with a frontier spirit, many indulged in legendary drinking and gambling bouts.

As with much of the West, San Francisco rode a boom-and-bust economy, and in 1855, the city suffered its first depression. To make matters worse, in just two years, six major fires swept the city. However, as the gold ran out, ranching, banking, and the construction trades helped diversify the region's economy. And then in 1859, another mineral discovery, this time of silver in nearby Nevada, returned the city to boom times.

The Comstock Lode—centered in Virginia City, Nevada—brought vast wealth to San Francisco. Enterprising San Francisco businessmen invested profitably in the Virginia City mines, and the city's merchants outfitted the miners.

Other forward-looking citizens helped build the transcontinental railroad, linking the city with the East Coast. These entrepreneurs built enormous mansions to celebrate their success, and the city center soon featured magnificent hotels, business blocks, and other emblems of a thriving economy. Tens of thousands of Chinese immigrants flocked to California to work on the railroad, and many settled in San Francisco.

The city suffered another economic downturn that lasted for most of the 1870s. Fortunately, San Francisco's diversified economy recovered, and by the 1880s the city was again vibrant. The harbor at San Francisco served a vast and fertile agricultural region, its shipping fleet delivering wheat and other agricultural products throughout the world. The city was the world's greatest whaling center for more than two decades, and whalers, cargo ships, ferries, yachts, and the city's fishing fleet kept the harbor always busy. To maximize ease of transport in San Francisco itself, a revolutionary cable car system carried citizens and visitors up the steep hills. And in 1894, to celebrate its good fortune, the city put on a world's fair, the Midwinter Exposition. Held in Golden Gate Park, the fair hosted more than 2 million tourists and city residents.

The year 1906 transformed the city. On April 18, at 5:12 A.M., a powerful earthquake shook San Francisco and the surrounding region. The earthquake, estimated to be 8.3 on the Richter scale, brought down many of the city's wood, brick, and stone buildings.

Devastating in its own right, the quake caused an even greater disaster: Several quake-caused fires coalesced to form a true firestorm, which reached temperatures upwards of 2,000 degrees F. With most of the city's water mains broken, firefighters faced a hopeless task, and after three days, San Francisco had lost the homes of 250,000 citizens—out of a population of 400,000—and 450 San Franciscans had died, either from the quake or fire. The elegant downtown, except for a handful of buildings, had been completely razed.

In photographs taken immediately after the fire, San Francisco's cityscape resembled those of Dresden and Hiroshima after the firestorms of World War II. With 490 blocks—2,800 acres—burned to the ground, San Francisco faced an enormous task. But with aid from around the world, the positive spirit of its citizens, and significant insurance settlements, the city soon emerged from its devastation. A large percentage of the buildings you see in today's San Francisco were built immediately following the disaster.

In 1915, San Francisco hosted another world's fair, this one known as the Panama Pacific International Exposition. The grand exposition celebrated both the opening of the Panama Canal and San Francisco's resurrection from the ashes. In what is now the Marina District, city engineers built a seawall and constructed the spectacular fairgrounds on sandy fill—setting the stage for more earthquake trouble in 1989.

As elsewhere, the Great Depression of the 1930s brought hardship to San Francisco. At the same time, public building projects funded through the New Deal provided jobs and created new Bay Area landmarks. Prominent among these projects were two remarkable feats of engineering, the Golden Gate Bridge and the Bay Bridge.

With the onslaught of World War II, San Francisco's fortunes revived. Bay Area shipyards began producing ships of all kinds for the war effort, and United States military outposts on the bay prepared to defend the city from enemy attack. The shipyards, working around the clock, produced many hundreds of ships, especially the huge cargo vessels known as Liberty ships. Luckily, the city's defenders never had to fire a shot.

Since World War II, San Francisco has seen some wild times. The 1950s and 1960s, for example, found the city—long known for its tolerance of the unconventional—a perfect testing ground for countercultural energies, with the rise of a Beatnik culture in the North Beach neighborhood and the Hippie explosion in the Haight-Ashbury. As before, the city has suffered the occasional economic downturn, most recently—and severely—in the late 1980s. And another major earthquake in 1989 damaged area freeways and turned the fill beneath the Marina District to jelly.

But with the coming of the 1990s, San Francisco is yet again the epicenter of a boom. This time, the treasures are virtual: the technological marvels—software, hardware, innovations on the Internet—concocted by the digital alchemists of nearby Silicon Valley. And at this writing, with the technology boom in full swing, the Bay Area's prospects for generating even more wealth seem limitless.

"The New Rome," one commentator calls San Francisco, and certainly all this wealth has given fresh energy to the city's cultural and civic institutions. City Hall and the city's opera house have undergone spectacular renovations; many of the city's museums have built, or are building, new homes; palm trees line the spruced-up Embarcadero; and a spanking new public library features state-of-the-art information technology. Already famous for its food, San Francisco now claims some 3,300 restaurants, more per capita than any other American city.

And San Francisco remains—with its compact size, stunning natural setting, richly textured urban fabric, and excellent mass transit system—perhaps the most congenial American city for those who love to walk.

walk 1

Downtown

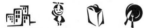

General location: The downtown and South of Market areas, in northeastern San Francisco.

Special attractions: Museums, downtown shopping, restaurants, theaters, urban landscapes, varied architecture, gardens.

Difficulty rating: Easy, flat, and entirely on sidewalks.

Distance: 2.5 miles.

Estimated time: 1.25 hours.

Services: Hotels, restaurants, restrooms, visitor information center.

Restrictions: Not wheelchair accessible. Dogs must be leashed and their droppings picked up. This is a densely packed urban setting; sidewalks are often jammed with people.

Downtown

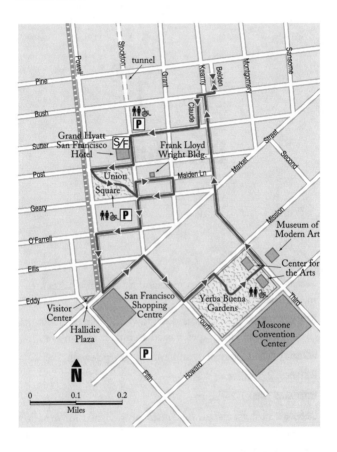

For more information: Contact the San Francisco Convention and Visitors Bureau.

Getting started: This walk begins at the main entrance of the Grand Hyatt San Francisco Hotel, located at 345 Stockton Street, 1 block north of Union Square.

(1) For freeway exits into San Francisco from the East Bay or the San Francisco Peninsula, refer to "Meet San Francisco" earlier in this book. From the intersection of Market, Third, Kearny, and Geary Streets, go north 2 blocks on Kearny. Go left on Sutter Street for 2 blocks. Turn right onto Stockton Street, and then take an immediate right into the entrance of the Sutter-Stockton Garage, one of the least expensive parking facilities close to Union Square.

(2) From the Golden Gate Bridge, continue on U.S. Highway 101 South and veer right onto the Downtown/ Lombard turnoff. Drive about 1 mile on Lombard Street, then turn right on Van Ness Avenue, and go 14 blocks. Turn left on Bush Street and go 9.5 blocks. One and a half blocks past the intersection of Bush and Powell streets, just beyond the bridge over the Stockton Street Tunnel, turn right into the entrance of the Sutter-Stockton Garage.

To reach the Grand Hyatt San Francisco Hotel from the Sutter-Stockton Garage, exit the garage onto Stockton Street, turn left, cross Sutter, and then cross Stockton to arrive at the hotel entrance.

Parking is also available at the Union Square Garage, which is beneath Union Square. Its entrance is on Geary Street. You will also find parking at the Fifth *&* Mission/ Yerba Buena Gardens Garage at Fifth and Mission Streets, 1 block south of Market Street.

Public transportation: Numerous San Francisco Municipal Railway (Muni) bus lines and Muni Metro lines run past or near Union Square. All Bay Area Rapid Transit (BART) lines stop at Market and Powell Streets, 3 blocks south of Union Square. AC Transit bus lines and Golden Gate Transit bus lines stop at the Transbay Terminal at Mission and First Streets, 1 block south of Market and 4 blocks east of Stockton. Contact Muni, BART, AC Transit, and Golden Gate Transit for information about schedules, fares, and accessibility.

Overview: Union Square is truly San Francisco's heart. This city's shoppers never abandoned their downtown for the seductions of suburban malls, and so the blocks around Union Square remain vibrant with mercantile high spirits. The retail mix includes art galleries, the city's most venerable hotels and department stores, and luxury specialty shops. Cartier, Armani, Gucci, Hermes of Paris, and the legendary Gump's are among them. You will also find a host of upscale mass retailers—Williams-Sonoma, Crate & Barrel, Banana Republic, Sur la Table, The Gap— several of which got their start in the Bay Area. Thriving without interruption since it was rebuilt after the 1906 fire, downtown San Francisco feels old-fashioned and up-to-the-minute at the same time, almost like the center of a great European city.

This truly urban walk guides you through downtown's retail mecca and into South of Market (SOMA, after New York's SoHo), the dynamic neighborhood that has metamorphosed from industrial district to key outpost in today's digital revolution. *Wired* magazine, the revolution's house organ, has its office here; and techno wizards work their magic in the district's renovated warehouses. SOMA is aswarm with trendy nightclubs and restaurants and the largest concentration of museums in the city. The stunning new San Francisco Museum of Modern Art—the second largest museum dedicated to modern art in America—is a must-see destination on this walk, and just across Third Street from the museum, the Yerba Buena Gardens offer multiple pleasures, from public art to sidewalk cafés to grassy knolls on which to recline after your long trek through crowded city streets.

The walk

➤Start at the front door of the Grand Hyatt San Francisco Hotel at the corner of Stockton and Sutter Streets.

➤Walk 1 block downhill on Stockton to Post Street. You will pass the circular fountain that San Francisco artist Ruth Asawa designed to "show what many hands working together can do." The scenes of San Francisco life depicted on this "folk monument" were modeled in bread dough—by visitors to San Francisco and by more than 100 children—and then cast in bronze.

➤Turn right onto Post and walk 1 block, passing Saks Fifth Avenue.

➤At Powell Street, turn left and cross Post to arrive at the northwest corner of Union Square. The tall building to your right, in the middle of this block of Powell, is the Westin St. Francis Hotel, a San Francisco landmark built in 1904 and restored after the 1906 fire. The cable car to Fisherman's Wharf passes the front door of the hotel.

➤Walk diagonally southeast through Union Square to the corner of Stockton and Geary Streets.

Union Square, in the midst of San Francisco's downtown shopping district, takes its name from pro-Union rallies held here during the Civil War. At the center of the square stands the Victory Monument, celebrating Commodore George Dewey's 1898 triumph over the Spanish fleet at Manila Bay. Street merchants and musicians station themselves at the corners of the square, and much of the year, you may chance upon an outdoor art show spread throughout this public space. Union Square is alive with that ubiquitous urban denizen, the pigeon, encouraged by the occasional bread-feeder.

➤Cross Stockton and turn left, walking one-half block uphill on Stockton to Maiden Lane.

To your left at the edge of Union Square is the kiosk for TIX Bay Area, which sells half-price, day-of-performance tickets (cash only) to theater, dance, and music events. Full-price, advance sale tickets are also available here. San Francisco's theater district lies on the other side of Union Square, bounded by Powell, Geary, Sutter, and Taylor Streets.

➤Turn right into Maiden Lane and walk 1 block.

Taking its name from its earlier history as home to the "maidens" of San Francisco's bawdy nightlife at the turn of the century, this is now a narrow, pedestrian-only street of quiet charm. Lined with small restaurants and elegant shops, it is a haven from the bustle around Union Square. Cafe tables spill out into the street, and tired shoppers recuperate with a salad, a crust of San Francisco sourdough bread, and a glass of wine.

The building at 140 Maiden Lane was remodeled in 1949 by master architect Frank Lloyd Wright. Faithfully restored in every detail in 1998, this architectural jewel—with its spiraling ramp—recalls on a much more intimate scale Wright's Guggenheim Museum of 1943. This landmark, now housing a folk art gallery, is definitely worth a visit.

➤Turn right onto Grant Avenue, and continue for one-half block until you reach Geary. You will pass several of the specialty stores that line Grant between Bush and Geary.

➤Turn right onto Geary and walk west, back toward Union Square. Britex Fabrics, midway along the block, boasts an inventory of textiles so large that it requires four floors to house it all.

➤At the corner of Geary and Stockton Streets, turn left and cross to the opposite side of Geary (to the entrance of Neiman Marcus) and then turn right to cross Stockton. The flower stands gracing these corners are a San Francisco tradition, adding sweetness and color to this crowded commercial intersection for more than 40 years.

➤Turn left onto Stockton and walk downhill, passing the entrance to Macy's San Francisco on your right and Macy's Men's Store on your left.

➤Turn right onto O'Farrell Street and walk 1 block to Powell.

➤Cross Powell, turn left, and walk downhill on Powell for 2 blocks to reach Market Street.

Located at the corner of Powell and Market Streets is the turnaround for the cable car that runs the steep hills between Union Square and Fisherman's Wharf. You will see people lining up to buy cable car tickets.

➤The Visitor Information Center of the San Francisco Convention and Visitors Bureau is also near this corner, below street level outside the Powell Street BART/Muni Metro station. Look for the signs for BART, and take the escalator leading down to the lower level of Hallidie Plaza. Cross the brick courtyard to the Visitor Information Center. After you have picked up an armload of brochures and had all your questions answered, return to the escalator and ride back up to the corner of Powell and Market. Look up and down Market Street to catch glimpses of the historic F Market Streetcar Line.

of interest

The Historic F Market Streetcar Line

Cable cars are one of San Francisco's signature attractions. But on this walk, you will also encounter the cable cars' lesser-known cousins, the brightly colored electric cars of the F Market Streetcar Line. Tracing its origins to 1860, this set of tracks has seen horse cars, steam engines, cable cars, and streetcars. Not just a piece of nostalgia, the F Market Line offers a delightful above-ground alternative to the subterranean Muni Metro lines that run beneath Market Street. As you walk along Market, you are bound to see the F Market cars or at least hear their distinctive purr.

A virtual inventory of disappearing electric streetcar systems worldwide, the F Market railway includes vintage cars from Australia, Italy, and Japan. Some of its historic streetcars sport the eye-catching color schemes of other American electric railways no longer in existence. Market Street Railway, a volunteer group founded in 1976, actively acquires and donates vintage streetcars to the San Francisco Municipal Railway (Muni). The volunteers also pitch in to help Muni restore and maintain its fleet of historic cars. Unlike San Francisco's famous cable cars, the F Market railway is powered—like some of the city's buses and the other San Francisco streetcar lines—by an overhead electrical cable.

The F Market Streetcar Line runs every day, from 6:15 A.M. to 12:30 A.M., along Market Street between the Transbay Terminal (at First and Mission Streets) and Castro Street. The F Line continues to expand; by the year 2000, it will travel all the way to Fisherman's Wharf, linking Upper Market, the central downtown shopping district, and the waterfront. For information about routes and stops on the F Market line, and other electric lines in the city, contact Muni.

➤Cross Market Street.

A few hundred feet to your right, at the corner of Fifth and Market Streets, is the entrance to San Francisco Shopping Centre, a vertical shopping mall with 90 upscale retail stores. It is noted for the escalator that spirals up through its central atrium.

➤Turn left onto Market and walk 1 block to Fourth Street.

➤Cross Fourth, turn right, and walk along Fourth for 1 block to Mission Street.

➤Cross Mission, turn left, and walk one-half block along Mission. When you reach the crosswalk in the middle of this block, look to your right to locate several openings into Yerba Buena Gardens.

➤Turn right into Yerba Buena Gardens and walk to the waterfall memorial to Dr. Martin Luther King, Jr., at the center of the gardens. Walk into the shade of the grotto behind the waterfall to read King's words, translated into the many languages of San Francisco's residents.

➤Walk up the ramp at the right of the waterfall to the upper level, which overlooks the garden and offers cafe seating on its terrace. From the balcony look toward the right edge of the garden to locate the large glass sculpture of a boat hull, *Seasons of the Sea Adrift*. Beyond and across Third Street, you will see the distinctive striped tower of the San Francisco Museum of Modern Art.

➤Walk down the ramp leading from the end of the balcony closest to Third Street.

➤Turn right, walk past the boat hull sculpture, and exit the garden onto Third.

➤Cross with the light to the entrance of the San Francisco Museum of Modern Art.

of interest

Yerba Buena Gardens

The 10 acres of the Yerba Buena Gardens count among San Francisco's most appealing open spaces. Here in the noisy midst of the South of Market area, you can find sanctuary from the urban hustle and bustle and, at the same time, enjoy a rich array of cultural offerings.

Set atop the giant Moscone Convention Center and just across the street from the San Francisco Museum of Modern Art, the Yerba Buena Gardens feature the Center for the Arts Galleries, Forum, and Theater. Other attractions include an outdoor stage, an ever-growing collection of public sculpture, and plenty of handsomely landscaped green space encircled by a paved esplanade.

A special feature is Reiko Goto's Butterfly Garden—on the northeastern edge of the esplanade—made up of plantings congenial to several species of butterflies native to the Bay Area. Another unique garden, on the upper terrace of the esplanade, honors San Francisco's 13 sister cities around the globe and features flowering plants from each. The centerpiece of the gardens—a stone and glass memorial to Martin Luther King, Jr.—offers a powerful message of peace and hope.

The Yerba Buena Gardens have been expanding since they first opened in 1993. The latest additions include a vast entertainment complex that features cinemas, restaurants, and shops and a state-of-the-art children's center that stretches over 4 acres. Also nearby, but not in the gardens, is the Ansel Adams Center for Photography.

The museum, relocated in 1995 from the Civic Center area to this site in South of Market, has been instrumental in extending the reach of San Francisco's downtown into this light industrial and warehouse district.

The museum's permanent collection focuses on modern and contemporary art; its schedule of temporary exhibitions nearly always includes a strong photography exhibit. The museum building, inspired by the Modernist tradition, was designed by Swiss architect Mario Botta. Particularly impressive are the spacious and skylit galleries on the top floor, and the bridge and circular stairway leading down from these galleries. The museum also has a fine gift shop with an emphasis on art books, as well as an excellent street-side cafe for the walk- or museum-weary.

➤Turn left—or if you are exiting the museum, turn right—and walk 1.5 blocks on Third toward Market.

➤Cross Market. You are now at the intersection of Kearny, Geary, and Market Streets.

➤Walk north on Kearny, away from Market Street, for 3 blocks.

➤Turn right onto Bush Street and then, after a short quarter block, turn left into Belden Place, one of the gathering spots in San Francisco's "European Quarter." Tucked into this tiny alley is a collection of smart French and Italian restaurants in a setting reminiscent of Montmartre in Paris. If the weather is good, you will witness, and perhaps partake in, a quintessential Parisian pastime: to linger at an outdoor table as the afternoon shadows grow long.

➤Exit Belden Place where you entered it, turn right, and return to the corner of Bush and Kearny.

➤Cross Kearny, turn left, and cross Bush.

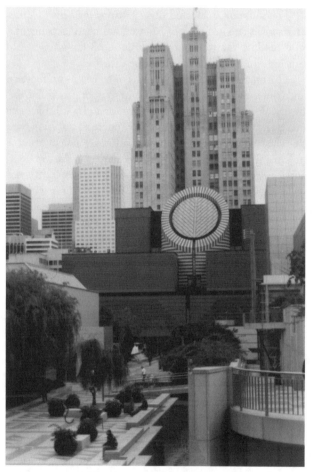

Directly across Third Street from Yerba Buena Gardens (foreground) stands the new San Francisco Museum of Modern Art.

➤Turn right onto Bush and, after one-quarter block, turn left into Claude Lane, another locus of the European Quarter and home to another small French restaurant.

➤Walk through Claude Lane to its opening onto Sutter Street.

➤Turn right onto Sutter and walk 2 blocks to Stockton. You will pass a number of well-known specialty retailers, including the flagship store of Banana Republic, as well as numerous art galleries. Many of the galleries are not on ground level; watch for their names on the brass name plates at building entrances.

➤Cross Stockton, turn left, and cross Sutter to return to the Grand Hyatt San Francisco Hotel and the end of this walk.

Chinatown

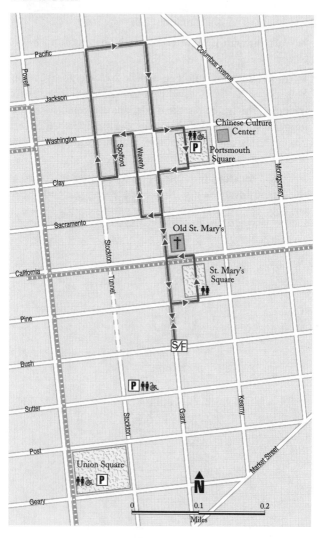

walk 2

Chinatown

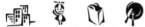

General location: In northeastern San Francisco, between the downtown shopping district and North Beach.

Special attractions: Chinese culture, historic architecture, shopping, restaurants, parks.

Difficulty rating: Easy, except that sidewalks are often extremely crowded. You will climb a few short hills.

Distance: 1.5 miles.

Estimated time: 1 hour.

Services: Restaurants, restrooms.

Restrictions: Not wheelchair accessible. Dogs must be leashed and their droppings picked up.

For more information: Contact the San Francisco Convention and Visitors Bureau, the Chinese Culture Center, or the Chinese Historical Society of America Museum.

Getting started: This walk begins at the gate to Chinatown at the junction of Bush Street and Grant Avenue.

(1) For freeway exits into San Francisco from the East Bay or the San Francisco Peninsula, refer to "Meet San Francisco" earlier in this book. From the intersection of Market, Third, Kearny, and Geary Streets, travel north 2 blocks on Kearny. Go left on Sutter Street for 2 blocks. Turn right onto Stockton Street, and then take an immediate right into the entrance of the Sutter-Stockton Garage, one of the least expensive parking facilities close to Union Square.

(2) From the Golden Gate Bridge, continue on U.S. Highway 101 South and veer right onto the Downtown/Lombard turnoff. Drive about 1 mile on Lombard Street, then turn right onto Van Ness Avenue, and go 14 blocks. Turn left onto Bush Street and go 9.5 blocks. One and a half blocks past the intersection of Bush and Powell Streets, just beyond the bridge over the Stockton Street Tunnel, turn right into the entrance of the Sutter-Stockton Garage.

To reach the Chinatown Gate from the Sutter-Stockton Garage, exit the garage onto Sutter Street, turn left, and walk a partial block downhill to Grant. Turn left onto Grant, and walk 1 block uphill to the corner of Bush and Grant.

Parking is also available at the Union Square Garage beneath Union Square and at the Portsmouth Square Garage at Kearny and Clay Streets in Chinatown.

Public transportation: San Francisco Municipal Railway (Muni) bus lines 2, 3, 4, 15, 30, 45, and 76 stop near the beginning of this walk. All Muni Metro and Bay Area Rapid Transit (BART) lines stop at Market and Powell Streets, 6 blocks from the Chinatown Gate. AC Transit and Golden Gate Transit bus lines stop at the Transbay Terminal at Mission and First Streets, 5 blocks from the beginning of this walk. Contact Muni, BART, AC Transit, and Golden Gate Transit for information about schedules, fares, and accessibility.

Overview: This stimulating walk takes you through San Francisco's most famous ethnic neighborhood. Chinatown—situated between downtown San Francisco and the bohemian enclave of North Beach—is second only to Fisherman's Wharf as a destination for visitors to the city by the bay.

This legendary community, where Chinese Americans maintain a clear cultural identity and many of the traditions of their homeland, is crowded and vibrant and endlessly intriguing. Here, along Grant Avenue and Stockton Street and in narrow alleys, you will find—in addition to the curio shops and restaurants aimed at tourists—the workaday world of Chinatown's inhabitants.

Well over 200,000 Chinese Americans live in San Francisco, and Chinatown is home to many of them. In recent years though, with Chinatown already overcrowded, recent Chinese immigrants from Vietnam and Hong Kong have settled in the Russian Hill, North Beach, Richmond, and Sunset districts. Even so, Chinatown remains the epicenter for Chinese culture in the Bay Area.

This walk leads you beyond Chinatown's usual tourist byways. Within these few blocks, you will discover tea houses and temples, fish and fowl markets, merchants in fresh vegetables and dried herbs, florists and fortune-cookie manufacturers, benevolent associations and banking houses. Give yourself plenty of time to take in the sights, sounds, smells, and tastes of Chinatown.

The walk

➤Start at the Chinatown Gate—complete with dragons—at the junction of Bush Street and Grant Avenue. The gate is just across Bush from San Francisco's tiny French Quarter and only a few blocks from downtown's Union Square.

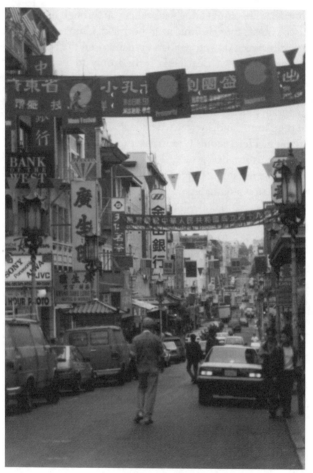

Chinatown is the vital heart of San Francisco's Chinese community.

➤Pass through the Chinatown Gate and head up Grant, the district's primary tourist thoroughfare. In this first block, you will pass many curio shops and art galleries.

➤Walk 1 block to Pine Street. Cross Pine and turn right, walking down Pine to the entrance of St. Mary's Square at mid-block. Turn left into this quiet mini-park, where you will find a public restroom, benches, lawns, and a monument. Created by noted sculptor Benny Bufano, the monument honors Dr. Sun Yat-sen, the reformer who led the 1911 revolution against the Manchu dynasty and established a modern republic in China.

➤Pass through St. Mary's Square and exit onto California Street. Take a left and walk up the hill to the corner of California and Grant.

Take a moment here to appreciate the striking church, Old St. Mary's Cathedral, directly across California. The brick walls and stone foundation of this landmark survived the 1906 earthquake and fire, and the remainder of the church was quickly rebuilt. St. Mary's is one of several Christian churches in Chinatown.

➤Cross California and continue down Grant, walking on the right side of the street. At the corner of Grant and Sacramento Street, look diagonally across to the large building on the corner. Note the colorful pagoda-like structure, with upturned eaves, at the top of this otherwise Western-style building, and the sign identifying it as the "Gold Mountain Sagely Monastery" run by the Dharma Realm Buddhist Association.

➤Cross Sacramento and turn left, heading up Sacramento for one-third block to Waverly Place. At the corner of Sacramento and Waverly (15 Waverly Place), you will see the Arts and Crafts–style brick First Chinese Baptist Church built in 1908 by architect G. E. Burlingame.

➤Take a right into Waverly Place, one of Chinatown's wonderful alleys and, since 1906, home to many of Chinatown's district and family associations. The people of Chinatown organized associations to aid their fellow immigrants in a variety of ways—everything from housing to burial costs. Family associations are organized around kinship, and the district associations benefit those who come from the same village or speak the same subdialect. Associations remain today a vital part of the Chinatown community.

In the first block of Waverly you will see several association headquarters. Note the Chinese-style decorative elements added to the top floors of these otherwise unassuming buildings.

➤Cross Clay Street and continue on Waverly. In the second block of Waverly, note on your left—at 125 Waverly Place—the Tin How Temple, a brightly decorated Taoist house of worship.

This temple with its intricately carved and gilded shrines honors Tien Hau, the Taoist Goddess of Heaven and the Sea, and many other gods and legendary figures. Born with a "heart full of compassion and good virtue," Tien Hau was "destined to be the savior of the mortals." The first Tin How Temple in San Francisco was built in 1852, making this the oldest Chinese temple in the United States.

➤Depart Waverly at Washington Street, turning left to ascend a partial block to Spofford Alley.

➤Turn left into Spofford, also known as New Spanish Alley. Many associations are located here, and as you walk through the alley, listen for the gentle sound—somewhere between a sigh and a rustle—of mahjongg tiles sliding across gaming tables.

Legend has it that Dr. Sun Yat-sen, first president of the Republic of China, lived in Spofford Alley when he came to San Francisco early in the 20th century. He was the guest of the Chee Kung Tong, also known as the Chinese Free Masons. Note the sign for this association at 36 Spofford Alley.

▶At the end of Spofford Alley, turn right onto Clay Street and walk uphill one-third of a block to Stockton Street.

At the corner of Stockton and Clay, look off to your left on Stockton. At 843 Stockton, you will see the brightly colored headquarters of the powerful Six Companies. Also known as the Chinese Consolidated Benevolent Association, the Six Companies is a kind of super-association responsible for taking care of the interests of the entire Chinatown community. To the left of the Six Companies headquarters is Chinese Central High School, one of several private schools in Chinatown devoted to instructing students in Chinese language and culture.

▶Cross Stockton and turn right to walk on the uphill side of Stockton for 3 blocks to Pacific Avenue.

Unlike Grant Avenue, Stockton was never intended to attract tourists. Instead, it serves as the main shopping street for Chinatown's residents. Here you will find many grocery stores, pastry shops, fishmongers, and poultry and meat markets, as well as herbal shops and acupuncturists.

Like Grant, Stockton is often extremely crowded, and as you walk, you will find yourself doing a kind of urban-density dance, twisting and turning, always looking ahead for an opening, that next bit of empty sidewalk. Do not forget to look up at the distinctive tops of buildings, or to take in the sights, sounds, and smells that make Chinatown a distinctive place. Venture into shops, stop for a moment at street corners to survey the bustling scene, and admire the skill and good humor with which the local residents navigate their neighborhood.

➤Take a right onto Pacific and descend Pacific 1 block to Grant. On this block, you will pass a Chinese-style housing project on your right. Built in the 1950s, these apartments are decorated in the three colors—red, green, and yellow—that signify happiness, longevity, and wealth in Chinese tradition.

➤Take a right onto Grant and walk 2 blocks to Washington Street.

➤Cross Washington and then turn left to walk down Washington. At mid-block, turn right into Portsmouth Square.

This historic park, today a community gathering place for Chinatown, was the plaza for the Spanish town—Yerba Buena, "good herb"—that predated San Francisco. In 1846, Captain John B. Montgomery claimed Yerba Buena for the United States and named the plaza for his ship, USS *Portsmouth*. The Chinese Culture Center is located across Kearny Street in the high-rise Holiday Inn. You may want to cross Kearny on the brick pedestrian bridge and take a few minutes to visit the cultural center's excellent art exhibits and bookstore. There is a city-owned parking garage on the lower level of Portsmouth Square.

➤Rest on Portsmouth Square's benches, admire its public sculpture, and if you are lucky, take in a performance of Chinese opera. When you are ready to move on, walk through the park onto Clay Street, turn right onto Clay, and head up the hill one-half block to Grant.

➤Turn left onto Grant and walk 4 blocks along this busy street to the Chinatown Gate and the end of this walk.

walk 3

North Beach

General location: In northeastern San Francisco, adjoining the Embarcadero, Chinatown, and Russian Hill.

Special attractions: Restaurants and coffee houses, shopping, urban landscapes, varied architecture, views, literary landmarks, public art, parks.

Difficulty rating: Somewhat difficult, with several steep hills.

Distance: 2 miles.

Estimated time: 1.5 hours.

Services: Restaurants, restrooms.

Restrictions: Not wheelchair accessible. Dogs must be leashed and their droppings picked up.

For more information: Contact the San Francisco Convention and Visitors Bureau or the North Beach Museum.

North Beach

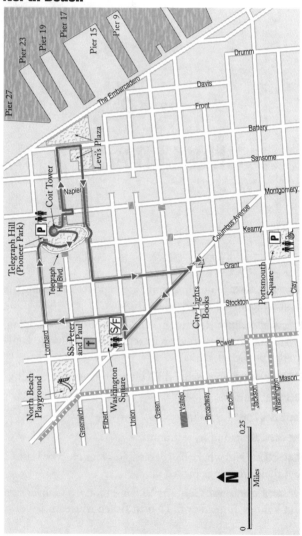

Getting started: This walk begins in Washington Square, at the corner of Union and Stockton Streets.

(1) For freeway exits into San Francisco from the East Bay or the San Francisco Peninsula, refer to "Meet San Francisco" earlier in this book. From the intersection of Market, Third, Kearny, and Geary Streets, go north 9.5 blocks on Kearny to Columbus Avenue. Turn left onto Columbus and go 4.5 blocks to Union Street. Turn right onto Union and go 1 block to the corner of Union and Stockton Streets.

(2) From the Golden Gate Bridge, continue on U.S. Highway 101 South and veer right onto the Downtown/Lombard turnoff. Drive about 1 mile on Lombard Street to Van Ness Avenue. Stay in the far left lane on Lombard, cross Van Ness, and continue straight ahead on Lombard for 1 block to Polk Street. Turn right onto Polk and go 3 blocks. Turn left onto Union Street and go 8 blocks to the corner of Union and Stockton Streets.

On-street parking in this neighborhood is always scarce and is time-restricted. The many small lots and garages are quite expensive; one of the more reasonable is the Vallejo Street Garage at 766 Vallejo. Parking is also available in nearby Chinatown at the Portsmouth Square Garage, on Kearny between Washington and Clay Streets. For a smooth beginning to your walk, we recommend taking a taxi or public transportation.

Public transportation: Buses 15, 30, 39, 41, and 45 of the San Francisco Municipal Railway (Muni) stop on Washington Square near the starting point of this walk. Contact Muni for information about schedules, fares, and accessibility.

Overview: This challenging walk—with its steep hill climbs—is one of San Francisco's most appealing. It starts out in the midst of exciting North Beach, at Washington Square, and quickly has you climbing. Soon, you will be savoring the views atop Telegraph Hill and the murals of Coit Tower—and then descending a famous San Francisco stairway through luxuriant gardens. After a quick breather near the waterfront, you will climb back up Telegraph Hill on another of those signature stairways.

The route then leads you down through the charming residential neighborhood on the slopes of Telegraph Hill and into the heart of North Beach, with its coffee houses, boutiques, galleries, and vivid street life. Here, the urban density is almost as intense as in neighboring Chinatown, but with a difference. Originally a neighborhood where European immigrants of many nationalities settled, North Beach was for many years an Italian enclave. Though it is now extremely diverse ethnically, North Beach retains a Mediterranean feeling. This quality is underscored by the numerous Italian espresso bars, *caffes,* delis, coffee roasters, and clothing stores that still line Columbus Avenue.

Like several other walks in this book, this walk showcases that particular San Francisco admixture of disparate cultures happily coexisting, of city life at its most exhilarating and natural beauty at its most breathtaking.

The walk

➤Start in Washington Square, at the corner of Union and Stockton Streets. Directly across from the starting point is Caffe Malvina, one of the classic coffee houses in the neighborhood. Another great spot to collect yourself is Mario's Bohemian Cigar Store Café, located 1 block away at the junction of Union Street and Columbus Avenue.

➤Leave Washington Square and cross Stockton Street to the front of Caffe Malvina. Take a left on Stockton.

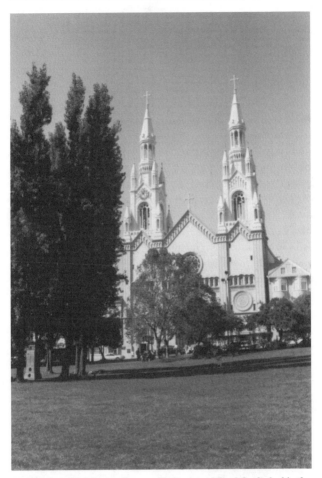

Visible from Washington Square, SS. Peter and Paul Cathedral is the spiritual home for many residents of North Beach's Italian community.

In mid-block, stop to gaze across Washington Square at SS. Peter and Paul Cathedral, one of San Francisco's most beautiful churches. Begun in 1922 and completed in 1939, SS. Peter and Paul is a Gothic Revival structure with a definite Italian feel, and it remains today the spiritual touchstone of North Beach's Italian community.

➤Walk 3 blocks on Stockton, crossing Filbert and Greenwich Streets.

You will pass the North Beach Athletic Club and North Beach post office, plus several restaurants, coffee houses, groceries, and bakeries. Liguria Bakery at the corner of Stockton and Filbert is particularly famous for its tasty focaccia, and often a line of customers snakes out the door. Peer into the charming courtyard of the handsome building at 1736 Stockton. Originally designed by renowned Bay Area architect Bernard Maybeck, the Maybeck Building today, appropriately enough, houses architects and designers.

➤At Lombard, the third cross street, turn right. You will see signs directing you up Lombard toward Coit Tower. Head up the steep hill for 2 blocks. Like most of the residential streets on Telegraph Hill, Lombard is home to a pleasing mix of new and old single-family dwellings, condominiums, and apartment houses.

➤Just beyond Kearny Street, near the start of Telegraph Hill Boulevard, Lombard stops abruptly at the edge of a cliff. Here you will find an overlook. Stop and admire the view of the Bay Bridge and the piers. On a clear day, you will be able to see Oakland and Berkeley across the bay.

➤To your right, you will see stairs ascending into the grove of cypress at the base of Coit Tower. Climb the stairs. They lead to a wide paved path that winds upward to the back side of Coit Tower. Walk around the tower to the front entrance.

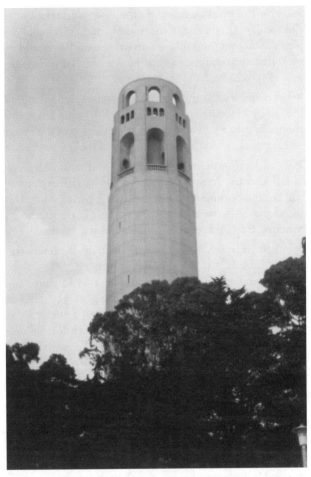

One of San Francisco's signature landmarks, Coit Tower crowns the peak of Telegraph Hill.

➤Circle the plaza surrounding the tower and take in the spectacular views, some of the finest in San Francisco. People from all over the world are drawn to Coit Tower, and on most days, you can hear a veritable United Nations of languages spoken here.

➤Enter the tower's front door to view the splendid murals created by 25 California artists during the 1930s. In the gift shop, you may purchase tickets to tour the top of the tower, where you can enjoy 360-degree views of the city by the bay.

➤Upon leaving the tower, turn right and cross Telegraph Hill Boulevard. At the street sign for Greenwich Street, you will see the beginning of the Greenwich Street stairs. Descend the brick steps through a verdant glade shaded by towering trees and past beautifully tended gardens.

➤When you reach Montgomery Street, the landmark restaurant Julius' Castle will be on your left.

Here you will find another great overlook. Pause and enjoy the extraordinary views. Unless it is a foggy day, you should be able to see—from various vantage points along the overlook—the marina at PIER 39 with lots of sailboats, the easternmost half of Alcatraz, Treasure Island, the Bay Bridge, and the apartment complexes and refurbished warehouses at the foot of the stairs. This is also the place to begin listening for the raucous chatter of the wild parrots of Telegraph Hill.

➤When you are looking straight across the bay at the white-columned pavilion on Treasure Island, turn right and walk alongside the overlook wall 30 paces or so on the lower half of the Montgomery Street loop. Watch for the sign that marks the beginning of the 300 block of Greenwich Street. At the sign, take a sharp left and descend the continuation of the Greenwich stairs.

➤Pass under a small overpass that belongs to the apartment house beside you. The stairs descend the hill, passing among modest bungalows, apartment buildings, and other private residences.

Again, you will descend through a series of lovely gardens. Watch for bushes of impatiens and roses, stalks of wild fennel, and expanses of nasturtium. Keep an eye out for the Telegraph Hill parrots, with their brilliant red heads and green bodies. Sometimes you can see them perched in the trees or on telephone lines, and you will almost certainly hear their harsh voices.

➤As you reach the bottom of the stairs, walk on Greenwich Street to its intersection with Sansome Street. Cross Sansome and continue 1 block farther on Greenwich to Battery Street.

➤Take a right onto Battery Street.

On your right, you will pass Il Fornaio, the Italian restaurant and bakery, a delightful place to refuel. Immediately beyond Il Fornaio, on both sides of Battery, is that urban oasis, Levi's Plaza. Here you will also find the corporate headquarters of Levi Strauss & Co., the well-known jeans manufacturing company founded in Gold Rush–era San Francisco; the lobby of the glass-fronted main building of Levi Strauss & Co. features a display that recounts the company's colorful history.

Take a breather in the plaza and savor the sounds of running water from the several fountains and the sight of public sculptures and the beautifully groomed lawns, which are a perfect spot for rest and recuperation.

➤When you are ready to continue your walk, exit Levi's Plaza through the broadest open area, to the left of the largest fountain, onto Sansome Street. Cross Sansome and head for the exposed cliff straight ahead, where you will find the beginning of the Filbert Street steps.

➤Climb back up Telegraph Hill on the Filbert Street steps. The steps will take you through another luxuriant garden, this one named for Grace Marchant, its founder and guardian spirit. As you climb, you will cross quaint Napier Lane, one of the last boardwalk streets remaining in the city.

➤When you return to Montgomery Street, look off to the left to see the elegant Art Deco apartment building at 1360 Montgomery—and the cutout of actor Humphrey Bogart in a third-story window. This elegant building was the setting for the 1947 film *Dark Passage,* starring Bogart and Lauren Bacall.

➤Cross the bottom half of the Montgomery Street loop, and climb the steps leading to the street's upper half. Cross Montgomery to the continuation of the Filbert Street steps. Head up the hill toward Coit Tower on yet another landscaped stairway, passing by a mass of bougainvillea vine and a sumptuous rose garden.

➤At the top of the stairs, veer left and walk on a driveway several feet to where Filbert meets Telegraph Hill Boulevard. Bear left, staying on the sidewalk, and descend Filbert 1 block to Grant Avenue.

➤At Grant, take a left and walk 3.5 blocks along this vibrant, almost always crowded shopping street known locally as Upper Grant. You will pass small neighborhood groceries, pizza joints, coffee houses, fine restaurants, bookstores, music emporiums, shops selling vintage and designer clothing, blues clubs, and the occasional purveyor of North Beach memorabilia. The Beat-era landmark Caffe Trieste—at Grant and Vallejo—offers the most powerful cappuccinos in the city.

North Beach: A Literary Place

City Lights Books is not the only literary landmark in North Beach, and Lawrence Ferlinghetti is not the neighborhood's only poet—though he currently serves as San Francisco's poet laureate. But City Lights and Ferlinghetti embody—and carry on—North Beach literary traditions that stretch back to the 1950s and even earlier.

Here, along these narrow streets and in the district's coffee houses and drinking holes, poets and fiction writers like Ferlinghetti, Allen Ginsberg, Gary Snyder, Lew Welch, and Jack Kerouac created a revolution in American letters. On one fabled night in October 1955, Ginsberg read his long poem "Howl" to an ecstatic audience at Gallery Six, and the San Francisco Poetry Renaissance was on, fueled by countercultural energies and the espresso of North Beach. Here, Beat poets and their followers—dressed in hipster black—celebrated a new freedom of language and lifestyle.

Today, you can still visit some of the legendary Beat hangouts: Enrico's, Vesuvio Café, Tosca Café, Caffe Trieste, and the U.S. Restaurant. Some, like the U.S. Restaurant, have been gentrified, their shabby charm stripped away in favor of a sleek nineties look, but the rest still, in atmosphere and attitude, hark back to that wilder time.

Poetry readings still happen in North Beach at City Lights and neighborhood cafés, and you will find alleyways and side streets named after this literary city's best-loved poets—Ferlinghetti, Kenneth Rexroth, Robert Duncan, Jack Spicer, Lew Welch—most of whom spent time in North Beach. "Pulse after pulse came out of North Beach from the fifties forward," wrote Gary Snyder in a famous essay, "that touched the lives of people around the world."

➤When you reach the corner of Grant and Columbus Avenues, continue downhill on Columbus for a partial block and cross Broadway. Turn right and cross Columbus. Turn left and make your way to the literary landmark directly ahead.

Situated at 261 Columbus, City Lights Books was the epicenter of the Beat explosion in San Francisco during the 1950s. Founded by poet Lawrence Ferlinghetti, this world-class literary bookstore remains a must destination for every book lover who visits the city. Besides offering many thousands of books on three floors—and staying open until midnight—City Lights maintains an active publishing program.

➤Once you have sated your bookish appetites, exit City Lights, turn left, and retrace your steps to Broadway. Then proceed up Columbus toward Washington Square. These long, densely packed 3 blocks represent the very heart of North Beach. You will encounter restaurants, Italian delis, curio shops, a seemingly endless string of atmospheric coffee houses—including our personal favorite, Caffe Greco—and hundreds of fellow pedestrians. Savor the sounds and smells of this bohemian pleasure ground. North Beach never fails to stimulate your nerve endings.

➤At the corner of Columbus and Union, cross Columbus and Union to Washington Square. Walk down Union to the corner of Stockton and the end of this walk.

walk 4

Russian Hill

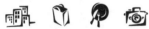

General location: In northeastern San Francisco, immediately north of downtown, west of North Beach, and south of Fisherman's Wharf.

Special attractions: Restaurants, shopping, urban landscapes, varied architecture, views of the city and the bay, public art, parks.

Difficulty rating: Somewhat difficult, with many steep hills and sets of stairs.

Distance: 3 miles.

Estimated time: 2.25 hours.

Services: Restaurants, hotels, restrooms.

Restrictions: Not wheelchair accessible. Dogs must be leashed and their droppings picked up.

Russian Hill

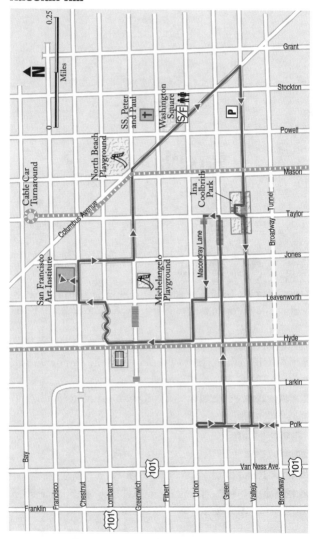

For more information: Contact the San Francisco Convention and Visitors Bureau.

Getting started: This walk begins at Washington Square in North Beach, at the intersection of Columbus Avenue and Union Street.

(1) For freeway exits into San Francisco from the East Bay or the San Francisco Peninsula, refer to "Meet San Francisco" earlier in this book. From the intersection of Market, Third, Kearny, and Geary Streets, go north 9.5 blocks on Kearny to Columbus. Turn left onto Columbus Avenue and go 4.5 blocks to the corner of Columbus and Union Street.

(2) From the Golden Gate Bridge, head south on U.S. Highway 101 South and veer right onto the Downtown/ Lombard turnoff. Drive about 1 mile on Lombard Street to Van Ness Avenue. Stay in the far left lane on Lombard, cross Van Ness, and continue straight on Lombard for 1 block to Polk Street. Turn right onto Polk and go 3 blocks. Turn left on Union Street and go 7.5 blocks to the corner of Union and Columbus Avenue.

On-street parking in this neighborhood is always scarce and is time-restricted. The many small lots and garages are quite expensive; one of the more reasonable is the Vallejo Street Garage at 766 Vallejo. Parking is also available in nearby Chinatown at the Portsmouth Square Garage, on Kearny between Washington and Clay Streets. For a smooth beginning to your walk, we recommend taking a taxi or public transportation.

Public transportation: Buses 15, 30, 39, 41, and 45 of the San Francisco Municipal Railway (Muni) stop on Washington Square near the starting point of this walk. Contact Muni for information about schedules, fares, and accessibility.

Overview: Russian Hill is one of San Francisco's finest residential neighborhoods. As you wander its steep, beautifully

landscaped stairways and streets, you will pass by some of
the few homes in this area of the city that survived the 1906
earthquake and fire. You will visit magical Macondray Lane,
a pedestrian street that has—through its residents' efforts—
become a garden wonderland. You will take a side trip to
the creative environs of the San Francisco Art Institute, with
its mural by famed Mexican painter Diego Rivera and the
sweeping views from Zellerbach Quadrangle. You will wind
down quirky Lombard Street, the famous series of sinuous
brick-paved switchbacks that forms one of the most popular attractions of the city by the bay. And you will truly test
your legs on some of this hilly city's steepest walkways.

The walk

➤Start in Washington Square, at the intersection of
Columbus Avenue and Union Street. Cross Columbus and
then turn left to cross Union Street. Then walk on Columbus for 2 blocks to Vallejo Street. In these 2 blocks, you will
pass classic North Beach restaurants, pastry shops, and coffee houses.

➤Turn right onto Vallejo. For the first block or so, you will
pass through the outer edge of Chinatown, but as you cross
Powell Street and begin the steep climb up Vallejo, you will
enter the district known as Russian Hill. You will pass block
after block of triple-decker flats, with their characteristic
bay windows and garages underneath. As you cross Mason
Street, you also cross the cable car tracks. The distinctive
buzzing you hear is made by the cables running just under
the rails.

➤Ahead on Vallejo you will see Ina Coolbrith Park, one of
the many beautiful stairway parks of San Francisco. The

park is named after a former California poet laureate; Coolbrith made her home in this once-bohemian neighborhood.

➤Take the set of stairs on the right side of Coolbrith Park and climb the steep, handsomely planted hillside. Quaint cottages in magical gardens, along with shingled apartment buildings, line the stairs. Look up and ahead to spot the ornate apartment house, with penthouse, at 945 Green Street, silhouetted against the sky.

➤At the first opportunity to leave the stairway, turn right onto the paved path that leads across the hillside past a set of park benches. In front of the benches, take in the cityscape spread out before you, especially the Bay Bridge, the Transamerica Pyramid, and the tall, dark Bank of America building.

➤Continue past the benches and mount the stone stairway that rises on your left and leads straight up the hillside. At the top of these stairs, go right and then left, as the path switchbacks up to Taylor Street.

➤Cross Taylor Street and continue up the stairs to the balustraded overlook at the top of Russian Hill. From the overlook you will see, from right to left, the rooftops of North Beach, the southern flank of Telegraph Hill, the piers at Fisherman's Wharf, and of course, San Francisco Bay with its sailboats, tugs, and tankers.

➤After the summit, descend to the ramp at the foot of this block of Vallejo. Notice the wonderful residences, ranging in age from early 20th century to brand-new, that line the street. Locate the stairways at the center of the ramp's headwall, and descend to Jones Street.

➤Cross Jones, and continue down Vallejo past more quintessential Russian Hill flats. As you cross Hyde Street, note the tracks of the Powell-Hyde cable car line, which runs between Union Square and Fisherman's Wharf.

➤Walk downhill for a total of 4 blocks to Polk Street and the friendly neighborhood shopping district of Polk Gulch.

➤Take a left onto Polk, walk 1 block to Broadway, cross Polk, and go right, walking back along Polk for 3 blocks to Union Street. Take in the wine shops, ethnic restaurants, coffee houses, fancy grocery stores, interior design and antique shops, and bookstores that make up this lively retail district.

➤At Union, take a right across Polk and then another right, returning down Polk 1 block to the corner of Green. Take a left onto Green, and walk up Green for 2 blocks to Hyde.

➤Cross Hyde and continue on Green for another 2 blocks to Jones Street. In the 1000 block of Green, between Leavenworth and Jones Streets, you will pass some of Russian Hill's oldest homes.

As chance would have it, this area escaped destruction during the 1906 earthquake and fire. Take special note of the octagonal house at 1067 Green, built in 1857, and the houses at 1045 and 1055 Green, built in 1866 and the 1880s, respectively. The block of flats at 1039-1043 Green, also built in the 1880s, was moved here after the fire. Another intriguing structure is the former firehouse at 1088 Green, built in 1907. These are private homes; please respect their owners' privacy.

➤Beyond Jones, walk a partial block on Green to another overlook offering great views of the Embarcadero, North Beach, and the Financial District. To the left of the overlook, descend a steep set of stairs to Taylor Street.

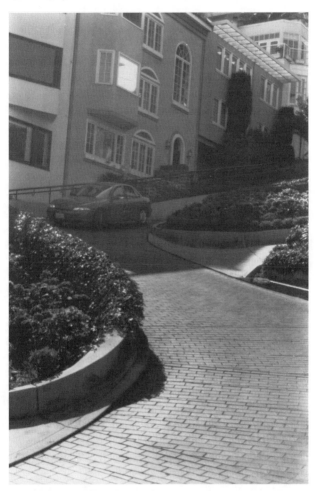

Brick-paved Lombard—perhaps the most famous street in the city— curves past classic San Francisco flats.

➤Turn left onto Taylor. Then after one-half block, turn left onto Macondray Lane. The block starts as a set of wooden stairs that rises precipitously from Taylor.

➤Climb the Macondray Lane stairs, and continue up the lane as it turns into a cobblestone, brick, and concrete pathway, between old and new homes. Ferns, an enormous eucalyptus, and fuchsia trees create a peaceful, grotto-like atmosphere right in the heart of one of San Francisco's most densely populated neighborhoods.

➤Cross Jones and walk another block on Macondray Lane.

➤Then turn right onto Leavenworth and walk one-half block to Union.

➤Take a left onto Union and walk 1 block to Hyde. At this corner, you will find the original Swensen's Ice Cream, a true Russian Hill landmark. With ice cream cone in hand, take a right onto Hyde and walk 3 blocks to Lombard Street.

➤Turn right onto Lombard and walk down the switchbacks of postcard fame.

Undoubtedly San Francisco's most famous street, Lombard was converted to switchbacks in the 1920s to lessen the steepness of the grade for automobiles.

➤At the bottom of the switchbacks on Lombard, fight your way through the crowds of photographers, turn left on Leavenworth, and walk 1 block. You will see Alcatraz Island directly ahead in the bay. At the corner of Leavenworth and Chestnut Streets, stop and take a look at the hillside garden the size of several city lots, just one-half block farther down Leavenworth.

➤Turn right onto Chestnut. Midway down the block, on the left side of the street, enter the building that looks like a Spanish monastery.

This is the San Francisco Art Institute, the city's finest art school. Walk though the courtyard, keeping to the left of a fountain stocked with colorful carp. At the far left of the courtyard, stop in the Diego Rivera Gallery to view the fresco—depicting the "design and construction of a modern industrial city"—painted by the great Mexican muralist in 1931.

➤After exiting the Rivera Gallery, continue down the corridor, away from the courtyard, to Zellerbach Quadrangle, the plaza atop a shiplike modern addition to this historic building. Note the smokestack-like skylights that look down into the institute's studios. From the quadrangle, you can enjoy some of the best views in the city. To the east, watch for Telegraph Hill and the Bay Bridge, and to the north, Fisherman's Wharf.

➤Exit the Art Institute where you entered it, onto Chestnut, and turn left. Continue downhill for one-half block.

➤Turn right onto Jones Street and walk 2 blocks.

➤Turn left onto Greenwich and walk 2 blocks to Columbus Avenue. You have left behind the relative tranquility of Russian Hill and are passing into the coffee-fueled excitement of the North Beach neighborhood.

➤Cross the cable car tracks and turn right onto Columbus. Walk 2 blocks to the corner of Columbus and Union. On your left will be Washington Square and the corner at which you started this walk.

walk 5

The Embarcadero

General location: On the bay waterfront in northeastern San Francisco, just north of the Bay Bridge.

Special attractions: Cafés and restaurants, bay views, access to ferries and bay cruises, historic district, and shopping arcades.

Difficulty rating: Easy, flat, and entirely on sidewalks.

Distance: 3 miles.

Estimated time: 1.5 hours.

Services: Restaurants, restrooms.

Restrictions: Wheelchair accessible. Dogs must be leashed and their droppings picked up.

For more information: Contact the San Francisco Convention and Visitors Bureau.

Getting started: This walk begins at the Ferry Building, located on San Francisco Bay just north of the Bay Bridge, where Market Street meets the Embarcadero.

(1) For freeway exits into San Francisco from the East Bay or the San Francisco Peninsula, refer to "Meet San Francisco" earlier in this book. From Interstate 80 West, take the Fremont Street exit and go to the intersection of Market, Fremont, and Front Streets. Cross Market and drive 3.5 blocks on Front to Clay Street. Turn right onto Clay and go 2 blocks to Drumm Street. Turn right onto Drumm and then make a left-hand turn into the garage beneath Four Embarcadero Center.

From U.S. Highway 101 North or I-280 North, go to the intersection of Market, Third, Kearny, and Geary Streets and drive 7 blocks on Kearny to Clay Street. Turn right onto Clay and go 6 blocks. Turn right onto Drumm and then make a left-hand turn into the garage underneath Four Embarcadero Center.

(2) From the Golden Gate Bridge, drive about 1.5 miles on US 101 South and then veer left onto the Marina exit. Follow the flow of traffic for 14 blocks along Marina Boulevard and Bay Street to the intersection of Bay and Van Ness Avenue. Continue on Bay for 11 more blocks, turn right onto the Embarcadero, and drive almost 1 mile. Turn right onto Washington Street and go 1 long block to Drumm Street. Turn left onto Drumm and go 1 block. Just after crossing Clay Street, make a left-hand turn into the garage underneath Four Embarcadero Center.

After parking, walk through Four Embarcadero Center at street level and then bear right through Justin Herman Plaza to Market Street. Turn left onto the pedestrian extension of Market and cross the Embarcadero to the Ferry Building.

The Embarcadero

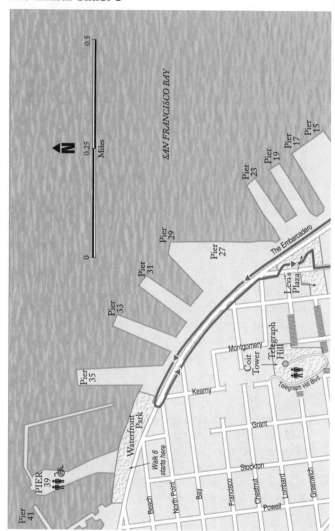

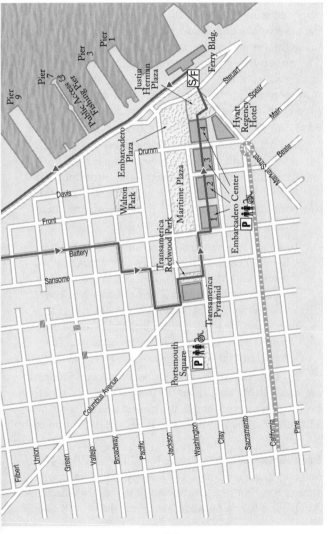

73

On Saturdays and Sundays, parking is available and quite inexpensive—in fact free with validation from any Embarcadero Center merchant—in the garages beneath the four office towers of the Embarcadero Center. However, on weekdays many garages in this busy commercial district fill by 8 A.M. The garages beneath Embarcadero Center, with more than 2,000 spaces, usually fill by 10 or 10:30 A.M. You can also stow your vehicle in a less crowded garage a bit farther away from Embarcadero Center. These include:

- Fifth & Mission/Yerba Buena Gardens Garage at Fifth and Mission Streets. From the garage, walk 1 block north on Fifth to Market Street. Muni buses 6, 7, 9, 66, and 71 run along Market to the Ferry Building. Muni Metro lines run underneath Market from the Powell Street Station to the Embarcadero Station near the Ferry Building.

- Portsmouth Square Garage on Kearny Street between Clay and Washington Streets. From the garage, walk downhill on Clay 6 blocks. Turn right onto Drumm Street, then turn left into Four Embarcadero Center, and walk through Embarcadero Center to Justin Herman Plaza. Bear right through the plaza to Market Street. Turn left onto the pedestrian extension of Market and cross the Embarcadero to the Ferry Building.

All garages listed above have wheelchair-accessible parking areas. If you are driving a van or RV, please note that height clearances are as follows: Embarcadero Center, 6' 6"; Fifth & Mission/Yerba Buena Gardens, 8' 1"; Portsmouth Square, 7'.

Public transportation: All Bay Area Rapid Transit (BART) trains and San Francisco Municipal Railway (Muni) Metro lines stop at the Embarcadero Station near the Ferry Building. Muni buses 6, 7, 9, 66, and 71 stop near the Ferry Building.

Golden Gate Transit bus lines and AC Transit bus lines stop at the Transbay Terminal, 5 blocks from the Ferry Building. Contact BART, Muni, Golden Gate Transit, and AC Transit for information about schedules, fares, and accessibility.

Overview: If you love the water and find waterfronts fascinating, this walk is sure to satisfy. And if you like to walk fast, the broad esplanade along the Embarcadero—Spanish for "pier" or "wharf"—is an excellent place to stretch your legs. Though runners and in-line skaters also make good use of this piece of pavement, it is rarely crowded.

But it is the water—San Francisco Bay—and the waterfront—the always-changing activity along the piers—that give this walk its salty savor. Times have changed and the port of San Francisco is no longer as active as it once was, but its piers are still in use, in new and old ways. A couple serve as headquarters for America's Cup contenders, while others have been retooled as classy waterside law and architects' offices or as space for off-price retail sales and temporary art expositions. A few are even devoted to their original use as dockside warehouses. You will see an old ferry boat that has made its last voyage and is now converted to a floating office building, as well as tractor tugs and pilot boats.

This is a wonderful place to walk on a foggy morning. Somehow the fog makes the scene more maritime, even more evocative of San Francisco's waterfront past: Foghorns sound in the distance, ghost ships slide silently by, the chop—invisible—slaps against the piers, a breeze moistens your face.

And when you are ready to leave the water, this walk leads you through San Francisco's first historic district, the elegant Jackson Square neighborhood with its fine antique shops and interior design studios. By a fluke, many of the structures here—including some built in the 1850s—survived the 1906 earthquake and fire.

The Embarcadero walk culminates, appropriately enough, in Embarcadero Center, an upscale shopping—and dining—complex extending over eight city blocks. The center stands just opposite the Ferry Building where this walk began.

The walk

➤Start at the front entrance to the Ferry Building—recognizable by its tall clock tower—where Market Street meets the Embarcadero. Ferries bound for the Marin County cities of Larkspur and Sausalito depart from the Ferry Building.

➤As you face the Ferry Building, odd-numbered piers run to the left; even numbers to the right. Turn left and walk on the esplanade that runs past Piers 1 through 45 along the Embarcadero.

Pier 1 is the terminus for commuter ferries departing for Oakland, Alameda, Tiburon, and Vallejo.

As you walk along the esplanade, look to your left at the skyscrapers of the Financial District. You may catch sight of a wisp of fog moving between two buildings, obscuring the top of one while its neighbor, just a block away, stands out in crisp detail.

➤At Pier 7, near the intersection of Broadway and the Embarcadero, is a long boardwalk—lined by old-fashioned street lamps—that extends out into the bay. Stroll to the end of the pier to feel the bay breezes, get a closer view of sailboats and ferries as they pass, and watch anglers try their luck.

From Pier 7, you can also see the ferryboat *Santa Rosa* docked at Pier 3, and you will have great views of the Bay

Bridge and Treasure Island. As you return to the esplanade, look up ahead to see the Transamerica Pyramid, a signature feature of the San Francisco skyline.

At Pier 15, headquarters for Bay and Delta Towing, you are likely to find a few tractor tugs, the small but powerful boats that literally push oceangoing vessels into their berths.

Near Pier 15, look at the skyline for a good view of Telegraph Hill, with Coit Tower at its peak and homes perched precariously on its steep slopes.

Along the esplanade, watch for the series of 10-foot-tall historical markers. The text and photos on these markers provide a real sense of what the waterfront was like, from the days of the clipper ships to the early 20th century. Also watch for the brief, vivid poems, many of them Japanese haiku, inscribed in the pavement underfoot.

➤When you are opposite Pier 23, cross the Embarcadero at the crosswalk to see a small historical marker with photos of the White Angel Jungle, a Depression-era soup kitchen that stood nearby. Here Lois Jordan, the "White Angel," fed "seamen without ships, longshoremen with no cargo to load, railroad men out of jobs, carpenters with nothing to build."

➤Just to the left of the White Angel marker, step into Levi's Plaza to glimpse the refreshing waterfall and shady, sloping lawns of this gracious urban park.

This small park lies adjacent to the corporate headquarters of Levi Strauss & Co., the well-known jeans manufacturing company founded in Gold Rush–era San Francisco in 1873. Beyond the park, in the Levi Strauss office complex, are several excellent restaurants and a large fountain, its waters cascading over granite and concrete ledges. The lobby of the glass-fronted main building of Levi Strauss & Co. features a display that recounts the company's colorful history.

➤Exit Levi's Plaza where you entered it, re-cross the Embarcadero, and turn left to continue your ramble around the eastern tip of the San Francisco Peninsula.

Just beyond Pier 23 sits a small jazz joint that has been on this spot since 1938 and gives a hint of the more modest wharfside architecture of days gone by.

A former Alcatraz prisoner told a friend of ours that one of the hardest things about being on the Rock was that, on balmy summer nights, music and laughter—from bars like this one—would float across the water, reminding him of the freedom he had left behind.

A little farther on, the last tall historic marker commemorates the old North Point-Lombard & Greenwich dock, the destination for clipper ships that rounded Cape Horn in the 1850s and 1860s. From this vantage point, the side of Telegraph Hill looks scooped out. In fact, it was. Ships from the East Coast would unload their cargoes in San Francisco, fill their holds with Telegraph Hill rock for ballast, and head back around the Cape.

Pier 35 is San Francisco's cruise ship terminal. As you pass, check the large sign on the face of the pier building to see which ships will be in port in the coming weeks.

➤Continue on the esplanade toward the stand of colorful flags that marks the beginning of Waterfront Park, which extends from Pier 35 to Pier 41.

➤Walk to the right of the flagpoles and up the boardwalk ramp that leads to a set of benches overlooking the water.

Stop a moment to gaze at Angel Island and the Richmond–San Rafael Bridge in the distance. Listen to the bay waters lapping against the piers. A bit farther on in Waterfront Park you will find several seating areas—set off by cobblestone paving and well-tended plantings—that are ideal for a picnic or a breather. And if you forgot to bring a lunch, there are plenty of restaurants on PIER 39, located midway in Waterfront Park and described in Walk 6, Fisherman's Wharf.

➤Return to the flagpoles at the beginning of Waterfront Park.

➤Cross the Embarcadero at the crosswalk near the flagpoles, turn left, and walk 3 blocks along the Embarcadero to its intersection with Battery and Lombard Streets.

➤Cross to the opposite corner of Battery. Here you will find the Fog City Diner, the exterior of which resembles a shiny chrome dining car. Stop to admire the old brick warehouse building across the street at 1333 Battery, with its handsome arched windows on several floors.

➤Walk on Battery just beyond the Fog City Diner to the entrance of Levi's Plaza.

➤Turn left into the park and follow the curved path through the park.

➤After passing the small fountain with water tumbling over different levels, turn right and walk back to Battery Street.

➤Turn left onto Battery and go 5 blocks to Pacific Avenue.

➤Turn right onto Pacific and walk 1 block to Sansome Street. Cross Sansome and then cross Pacific.

➤Go 1 block on Sansome to Jackson Street. Notice the distinctive building facades at 710 and 712 Sansome.

➤Turn right onto Jackson and walk 1 block along this charming tree-lined street with its fine antique stores, decorator shops, and oriental rug and vintage poster dealers.

You are now at the heart of the Jackson Square Historic District. As fate would have it, this neighborhood escaped the 1906 fire. Today it offers a rare glimpse into Gold Rush–era San Francisco. Be sure to look up at the ornate facades—

constructed of cast stone and cast iron—along this block. Especially notable is the Hotaling Building, originally home to a wholesale liquor company, at 451-455 Jackson.

➤Turn left onto Montgomery Street and walk 1 block to Washington Street.

Note the historic Belli Building at 722-728 Montgomery. This was the site of the founding of freemasonry in California in 1849, and until recently the building held the law offices of famed criminal defense attorney Melvin Belli. Built in 1851, it is believed to be the oldest surviving building in downtown San Francisco. This structure was also known as the Genella Building, after original owner Joseph Genella, purveyor of glassware and fine china. It was home to many artists' studios between the 1880s and the 1930s.

➤Cross Washington and enter the lobby of the Transamerica Pyramid. Wheelchair-accessible doors are located on the Washington Street side of this corner of the Pyramid.

➤Walk through the lobby, which features art exhibitions, to the Virtual Observation Deck that lies at the back, beyond the telephones and elevators.

Here, four screens show views—transmitted from scopes mounted on top of the Pyramid—to the north, south, east, and west. Feel free to move a scope's orientation and zoom in to see all quadrants of San Francisco—in real time and astonishing detail. Kids will love the Virtual Observation Deck.

➤Exit the Transamerica Pyramid the same way you entered it. Go right on Washington for one-half block to the entrance of Transamerica Redwood Park.

➤Turn right and walk through the park to the opposite entrance on Clay Street, just beyond the "frog pond" fountain. This park's 80 solemn redwoods—transplanted from

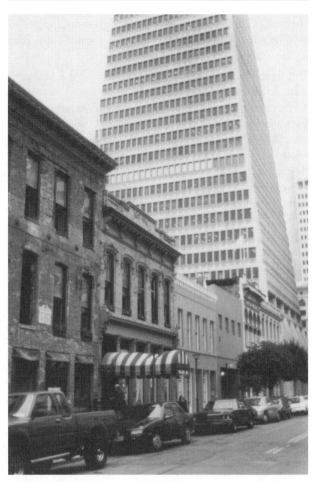

One of San Francisco's oldest buildings, built in 1851, is dwarfed by another city landmark, the Transamerica Pyramid.

the Santa Cruz Mountains—its flowers, greenery, and whimsical bronze sculptures create a breathing space at the edge of the Financial District.

➤Exit the park onto Clay and turn left. Go 1.5 blocks to Battery Street.

Near the corner of Clay and Sansome Streets, you will pass a bronze plaque that marks a site linking today's Financial District to its mercantile past. During the Gold Rush, when San Francisco's shoreline came up to Montgomery Street, the ship *Niantic* graced this location. It was no longer used as a seafaring vessel but instead as offices, stores, and a warehouse in the fast-growing young city.

➤Cross Clay, cross Battery, and proceed a partial block on Battery to the entrance of One Embarcadero Center. A ramp for wheelchairs is located on the right side of the entrance area.

Embarcadero Center extends over eight city blocks. The lower three levels of its four office towers are home to more than 125 shops and restaurants. You will find escalators at the center of each building. Wheelchair-accessible elevators are located adjacent to the elevators to the parking garage, and there are wheelchair-accessible restrooms on the lobby level of each building. On the 41st floor of One Embarcadero Center is an observation deck called SkyDeck. Besides 360-degree views of all of San Francisco, SkyDeck offers interactive computer kiosks that interpret the history and cultural life of the Bay Area. The SkyDeck ticket booth is located on the street level of One Embarcadero Center.

➤Walk through One Embarcadero Center toward its exit on Front Street, following signs to Two Embarcadero Center.

➤Continue to walk through the shopping complex, following signs to Three Embarcadero Center and Four Embarcadero Center. Exit Four Embarcadero Center onto Justin Herman Plaza.

➤Bear right along the plaza, heading toward the Hyatt Regency Hotel and Market Street.

Justin Herman Plaza is a much-used public space. On warm days people relax near the fountain or at the sidewalk tables on the terrace. During the summer, Embarcadero Center hosts outdoor concerts; in winter, an outdoor ice skating rink adds a snowbelt touch to this temperate setting. Street merchants do a brisk business on the Market Street side of the plaza, especially during the holiday season. Saturday and Sunday mornings the Ferry Plaza Farmers Market brings the place alive. Shop here for some of the Bay Area's best organic produce and artisanal cheeses and breads.

Justin Herman Plaza also is home to two public sculptures. The *Vaillancourt Fountain* dominates the landscape at the north end of the plaza. By Montreal sculptor Armand Vaillancourt, the fountain is made up of 101 boxes of precast aggregate concrete. At the other end of the plaza, near the Hyatt Regency, check out the bright metal sculpture called *La Chiffonnière*. By world-renowned French artist Jean Dubuffet, *La Chiffonnière* ("Rag Woman") is constructed of stainless steel with linear tracings of black epoxy.

➤Walk past the Hyatt Regency to Market Street. Turn left onto the pedestrian extension of Market and cross the Embarcadero to the Ferry Building and the end of this walk.

walk 6

Fisherman's Wharf

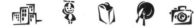

General location: On the bay waterfront in northeastern San Francisco, just north of North Beach and Russian Hill.

Special attractions: Museums, PIER 39 shopping arcade, cafés and restaurants, coastline, floating national historic park, sea lions, access to ferries and bay cruises.

Difficulty rating: Easy, flat, and entirely on sidewalks.

Distance: 2.5 miles.

Estimated time: 1.25 hours.

Services: Parking, restaurants, restrooms.

Restrictions: Wheelchair accessible. Dogs must be leashed and their droppings picked up.

For more information: Contact the San Francisco Convention and Visitors Bureau.

walk **6**

Getting started: This walk begins at the front entrance to PIER 39, on the Embarcadero between Beach and Jefferson Streets.

(1) For freeway exits into San Francisco from the East Bay or the San Francisco Peninsula, refer to "Meet San Francisco" earlier in this book. From Interstate 80 West, take the Harrison Street/Embarcadero exit—the first left exit after crossing the Bay Bridge. Turn right onto Harrison Street, go 4 blocks, then turn left onto the Embarcadero, and continue about 1.5 miles to PIER 39. From the San Francisco Peninsula, take U.S. Highway 101 North to I-80 East and then take the Fourth Street exit—or take I-280 North to its Sixth Street exit—and then go east on Bryant Street almost 1 mile. Turn left onto the Embarcadero and continue almost 2 miles to PIER 39.

(2) From the Golden Gate Bridge, drive about 1.5 miles on U.S. 101 South and then veer left onto the Marina exit. Follow the flow of traffic for 14 blocks along Marina Boulevard and Bay Street to the intersection of Bay and Van Ness Avenue. Continue on Bay for 11 more blocks, turn left onto the Embarcadero, and go 2.5 blocks to PIER 39.

On-street parking is extremely difficult in the Fisherman's Wharf area, and parking garages are quite expensive. Parking is available at the PIER 39 Garage directly across the Embarcadero from PIER 39; at the Anchorage on Jones Street between Beach and North Point Streets; at Ghirardelli Square on Beach between Polk and Larkin Streets; and at numerous street-level parking lots in the area.

All the parking garages listed above have wheelchair-accessible parking areas. If you are driving a van or RV, height clearances are as follows: PIER 39, 6'8"; the Anchorage, 6'8"; Ghirardelli Square, 6'.

Note: To avoid Fisherman's Wharf congestion, you may prefer to park in the free lots at Fort Mason Center or along the Marina Green—for the Marina Green, see map on

Fisherman's Wharf

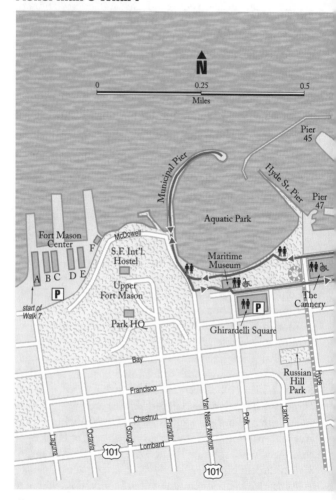

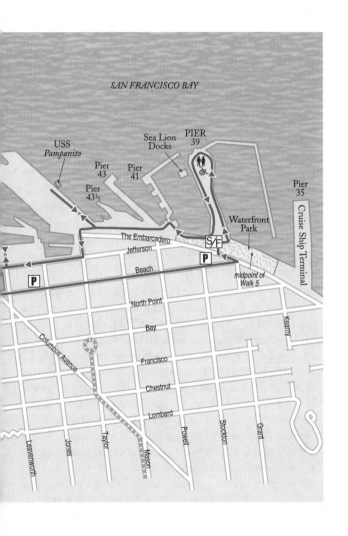

SAN FRANCISCO BAY

USS *Pampanito*

Pier 43

Pier 41

Pier 43½

Sea Lion Docks

PIER 39

Pier 35

The Embarcadero

Jefferson

Beach

North Point

Bay

Francisco

Chestnut

Lombard

Waterfront Park

Cruise Ship Terminal

S/F

midpoint of Walk 5

Columbus Avenue

Leavenworth

Jones

Taylor

Mason

Powell

Stockton

Grant

Kearny

page 100—and reverse this walk by starting at the Municipal Pier in Aquatic Park. To reach the pier from Fort Mason Center, climb the steep stairs—not wheelchair accessible—leading out of the Fort Mason Center parking lot opposite Building E. At the top, turn left and take the brief and delightful walk along McDowell Street as it rounds the hilly headland between Fort Mason Center and Aquatic Park and descends to the pier.

Public transportation: San Francisco Municipal Railway (Muni) bus 32 runs from the downtown area to PIER 39. Buses 15 and 42 run from downtown to within a few blocks of PIER 39. Bus 30 runs from downtown to North Point Street, 1 block south of Aquatic Park. Buses 15, 32, and 42 are wheelchair accessible; bus 30 is not. Both the Powell/Hyde and Mason/Taylor cable car lines run to the Fisherman's Wharf area. Contact Muni for information about schedules, fares, and accessibility.

Overview: Fisherman's Wharf is the number-one destination for visitors to San Francisco—and with good reason. The wharf stretches from carnival-like PIER 39 to the curving municipal pier at Aquatic Park. In between, you will find a host of other attractions, enough to engage your interest for hours on end: the Hyde Street Pier, a floating national park that is home to the world's largest collection of historic ships; "Fish Alley" and the city's fishing fleet; more than 100 restaurants, many serving seafood caught fresh that day; the brick factories converted to shopping meccas known as the Cannery and Ghirardelli Square; and the always fascinating San Francisco Maritime Museum.

Though this walk is not particularly long or strenuous, we recommend allowing plenty of time to take in all the attractions. For the best possible experience, we suggest starting out early in the morning. The wharves are less crowded then, and there is likely to be fog, at least enough to add a dash of romance to this already enchanting scene.

Fisherman's Wharf remains the home of San Francisco's fishing fleet—dominated today by Italian Americans, as it has been since the turn of the century—but the fishing industry is much smaller than in years past. Today tourism is the real business of Fisherman's Wharf, and certainly the PIER 39, Cannery, and Ghirardelli shopping and dining arcades are a powerful draw. But we most love the attractions that celebrate San Francisco's seagoing past: the floating museum at Hyde Street Pier and the San Francisco Maritime Museum in Aquatic Park.

Enjoy it all, but in the midst of the tourist frenzy, take a deep breath, gaze out into the bay, and imagine the days when fishing boats, clipper ships, paddle tugs, and schooners swarmed these fabled waters.

The walk

➤Start in front of PIER 39 on the Embarcadero, at the benches beneath the pedestrian bridge spanning the Embarcadero between PIER 39 and its parking garage. With the Embarcadero on your right, walk straight ahead past the main entrance to PIER 39. On your left, you will see PIER 39's wild array of signs, overhead stairways, and small shops.

➤Continue past the main mall area of PIER 39 and take a left at the next opportunity, just before the Underwater World Aquarium building.

Walk through the wide passageway to the marina.

➤Turn left and walk counterclockwise around the perimeter of PIER 39, following the signs reading "Follow Salty." At the end of PIER 39, you will find an expansive view of

San Francisco Bay, including Alcatraz Island with Angel Island behind it, Treasure and Yerba Buena Islands, and the Bay Bridge. Stop for a moment and watch the activity on the bay.

One morning we witnessed an astonishing maritime dance during the short ten minutes we stood here. A cruise ship—immense as a floating city block—glided into the cruise ship terminal, pushed by a tiny tractor tug. A seaplane landed in the wake of the cruise ship, and tour boats chugged out to Alcatraz. A flock of pelicans flew past, adding to the magic of the moment.

➤Continue around the end of PIER 39, and bearing left, walk along the railing on the west side of the PIER 39 complex.

Here you will find a noisy pride of sea lions—as many as 200 of them—lolling on old wooden docks. You will hear them barking before you round the corner, and you will certainly smell them. Watch as solitary sea lions swim up and struggle to find a place on the already overcrowded docks. Most kids and nature lovers find the sea lions of Fisherman's Wharf endlessly fascinating.

➤Continue along PIER 39's perimeter, walking past the sea lions toward the Embarcadero. At the first opportunity, turn right and walk alongside the railing at the docks of the Blue & Gold tour boat fleet.

➤Just past the tour boat harbor, turn right and walk on the lamppost-lined boardwalk that stretches out into the bay just before you reach Pier 41. In a seating area on the right side of the boardwalk, in what looks like a large planter, you will find a 12-foot-square relief map. The map depicts—in considerable detail— the bay and the San Francisco Peninsula, the East Bay, and the North Bay.

➤Return down the boardwalk, turn right, and walk past Pier 41, the terminal for the ferries to Alcatraz Island and Angel Island, as well as for several bay tour boats.

➤Just beyond Pier 41, walk along the sidewalk that is marked off with a series of short wooden pilings linked by a heavy chain. This sidewalk parallels the continuation of the Embarcadero, although at this point the roadway begins to look more like a parking lot.

➤Just before you reach the main entrance to Pier 45, watch for the banner on the right that announces: "WWII Submarine National Historic Landmark." Walk out on Pier 45 to view the USS *Pampanito*, a World War II fleet submarine open for touring. As you walk along the pier, note the signs—surely unique in a tourist area— that warn you not to sit on the torpedoes alongside the wharf building.

➤Return along Pier 45, turn right, and walk about 100 feet to the intersection of Taylor Street with the end of the Embarcadero.

➤Turn left to cross the Embarcadero, and walk on Taylor for 1 short block to Jefferson Street. On the right side of Taylor, colorful outdoor stalls sell whole crabs as well as seafood cocktails that you can savor as you walk along.

➤Turn right onto Jefferson and walk 2 blocks to Leavenworth Street.

On your right, you will pass the Jefferson Street lagoon, where commercial fishing boats dock after selling their catch. These tightly packed docks are a jumble of white boats— with names like *Dixie, Mayflower,* and *High Hopes*—trimmed in cheerful tones of green, blue, yellow, and red. Most are weatherworn, and a few appear barely seaworthy. This appealing harbor is lined by seafood restaurants with nice big windows. Along Jefferson Street, you will also find shops that supply the fishing fleet with serious nautical gear: brass compasses, fish knives, and all manner of seagoing hardware.

➤At Leavenworth, turn right onto the wide alleyway known as "Fish Alley." Starting at dawn, fishing boats pull in here to deliver their harvests of shrimp, crab, squid, salmon, sole, and sea bass.

➤Return to the corner of Jefferson and Leavenworth, cross Jefferson, and turn right.

As you walk along the more crowded parts of Fisherman's Wharf—like Jefferson Street—keep an eye out for the notorious "jumping bush." For the past several years, a street performer costumed in leafy twigs has crouched at the edge of the sidewalk, looking just like a decorative bush. When an unwary tourist passes, he leaps up, throws out his arms, and scares the living daylights out of the unlucky passerby. Amused onlookers gather some distance away, watching this scene unfold again and again.

➤Following Jefferson, go one-half block to the wheelchair-accessible entrance—marked Cannery North—to the Cannery. An elevator is located just inside the Cannery North entrance, on the right.

This old brick building, formerly a Del Monte packing plant, now houses an eclectic group of restaurants and stores, many of which have an international flavor. On the third floor is the Museum of the City of San Francisco. This small gem of a museum offers well-designed exhibits on the history of the Bay Area, including both the 1906 and 1989 earthquakes. The Cannery's street-level courtyard is quite pleasant, planted with olive trees and other non-leaping shrubs. Weather permitting, live music is performed here year-round.

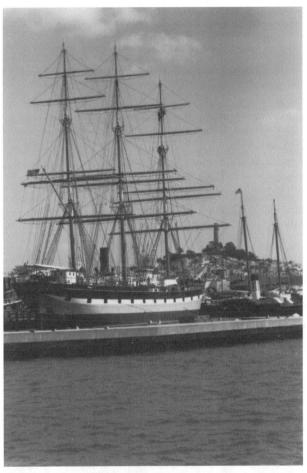

The masts of the great sailing ship, Balclutha, *loom above the Hyde Street Pier and its flotilla of historic boats.*

A Floating Museum

From a sidewheel ferry to a scow schooner, a square-rigged sailing vessel to steam-driven tugs, the "floating museum" officially known as the San Francisco Maritime National Historical Park is a must-see attraction along Fisherman's Wharf.

Walk out on the Hyde Street Pier to visit the historic ships that make this park unique. Here you will find the towering three-masted sailing ship, *Balclutha;* a pair of ocean-going tugs, *Eppleton Hall* and *Hercules;* the last San Francisco Bay scow schooner still floating, *Alma;* the *Eureka,* a powerful early-20th-century ferry; and a schooner used in the lumbering trade, *C. A. Thayer*.

The three largest vessels—the *Balclutha, Eureka,* and *C. A. Thayer*—are open for touring, and you will be able to walk their decks and peek into their cabins and holds. Sailors and shipwrights regularly demonstrate seafaring skills here, and the many excellent exhibits help you imagine what San Francisco's waterfront was like over the past 100 years.

Be sure to visit the San Francisco Maritime Museum at the foot of Polk Street, another key part of this national park. The museum features a Steamship Room, many nautical artifacts, and special exhibits on whaling, the China trade, and the days of the Gold Rush, when scores of captains and crews abandoned their ships in San Francisco harbor and headed for the goldfields. You may also want to stop in at the J. Porter Shaw Library, at Fort Mason Center, Building E. It features 12,000 volumes on maritime subjects.

For those who want to learn even more, the national park regularly offers classes, talks, demonstrations, and tours. Learn about battleships, pirates, and the crafting of wooden boats. And if you love the music of the sea, the park sponsors monthly concerts that feature ballads, sailor's songs, chanteys, and nautical fiddle airs.

➤After exploring the Cannery, exit onto Jefferson Street and walk to the end of the block at Hyde Street.

➤Turn right and cross Jefferson. Straight ahead lies the Hyde Street Pier, home to a "floating" San Francisco Maritime National Historical Park. You will almost certainly want to visit this intriguing collection of historic ships—and the wonderful bookstore featuring all tomes nautical.

➤Turn left onto Jefferson to enter Aquatic Park, a wonderful public space that includes Victorian Park (designed by famed landscape architect Thomas Church), the San Francisco Maritime Museum, the Hyde Street cable car turnaround, and a curving municipal pier that embraces a quiet cove.

As you enter Aquatic Park, note the two old buildings on your right. These are the clubhouses of two legendary swimming and boating clubs that date from before the turn of the century, the South End Rowing Club and the Dolphin Swimming and Rowing Club. Club members swim year-round in the bracing waters of Aquatic Park. If you spot a bright orange swim cap bobbing in the water, you have seen a club swimmer at play.

➤Staying close to the water, walk on the promenade around the cove. You will pass a sandy beach, a large set of concrete bleachers facing the cove, and the San Francisco Maritime Museum. This wonderful Streamline Moderne building was modeled after an ocean liner of the 1930s.

➤Just after passing the museum and another, smaller set of concrete bleachers, follow the asphalt ramp that slopes gently up and away from the water toward a tree-lined street—the quiet surprise ending of the otherwise congested thoroughfare of Van Ness Avenue.

➤Turn right onto the sidewalk that borders Van Ness Avenue and walk for 1 block to the intersection of Van Ness and McDowell Street and the beginning of the municipal pier.

➤Walk out onto the pier. This is a great way to get out on the bay without a boat, and the pier offers the best landlubber's view of Alcatraz Island, as well as splendid views of the Golden Gate Bridge and the Marin Headlands.

In addition to other promenaders, you will probably see some people fishing or crabbing off the pier. If you are strolling via wheelchair, we recommend using the wide center roadway. The lanes on either side of the roadway—created by high concrete curbs—get uncomfortably narrow in a few spots, and you cannot get out of these lanes until the very end of the pier.

➤Return to the start of the pier and walk straight ahead on the sidewalk at the left of Van Ness Avenue for about 1 block. Pass the whimsically round public restroom with exterior stairs and an observation deck for viewing the cove.

➤Continue past the gently sloping ramp that you used previously to reach Van Ness Avenue. Do not descend this ramp.

➤Turn left onto the next paved pathway, which is quite wide and slopes downward toward the Maritime Museum past a series of benches backed by a hedge and a line of quirky acorn-topped stone ornaments.

To your right, you will notice a covered playing court for bocce ball and groups of men in serious pursuit of this Mediterranean sport. The two tall, curving condominium towers behind the bocce ball courts are referred to by locals as the "Buck Teeth on the Bay."

➤Walk to the front entrance of the Maritime Museum on Beach Street.

➤Proceed up the ramp that leads to the polished chrome front doors to enter the museum.

The San Francisco Maritime Museum is a must for fans of author Patrick O'Brian or anyone entranced by the lore of the sea. Portions of the museum's collection—ranging from models of clipper ships to actual fishing boats—are always on display, and fascinating rotating exhibits focus on San Francisco's rich maritime heritage. Created as a recreation center and bathhouse by the Works Progress Administration during the 1930s, the museum features ocean-inspired murals in the lobby and cheerful mosaics of sea creatures on the balcony overlooking Aquatic Park.

➤Exit the museum through its front entrance and turn left onto Beach Street.

On your right, between Polk and Larkin Streets, is another shopping complex restored from an early-day factory. Ghirardelli Square was originally a woolen mill and then a chocolate factory. Now it is packed with specialty shops, restaurants with splendid bay views, and of course, San Francisco's own Ghirardelli Chocolate.

The wheelchair-accessible entrance to Ghirardelli Square is on North Point Street, 1 fairly steep block up Larkin or Polk from Beach. There is no wheelchair access from the sidewalk along Beach.

➤Walk along Beach for 2 blocks to Hyde Street. Beach Street is often lined with street artists and craftspeople selling their wares. As you near Hyde, you will pass the Hyde Street cable car turnaround on your left.

➤At the corner of Beach and Hyde, cross Beach and then cross Hyde.

On the southwest corner is the Buena Vista Café, a San Francisco landmark known as the place where, in 1952, the first Irish coffee in America was served.

➤Continue on Beach for 7 blocks until you reach the Embarcadero at PIER 39 and the end of this walk.

walk 7

Marina Green

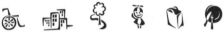

General location: Along the bay shoreline in north-central San Francisco, roughly equidistant between the Golden Gate Bridge and the Bay Bridge. Includes part of the Golden Gate National Recreation Area (GGNRA).

Special attractions: Museums, restaurants, marina and bay views, great strolling.

Difficulty rating: Easy and flat; on sidewalks except for a side trip to the Wave Organ.

Distance: 3 miles. Side trip adds 0.8 mile.

Estimated time: 1.5 hours, or 2 hours with side trip.

Services: Parking, restaurants, restrooms, visitor information center.

Restrictions: This walk is wheelchair accessible, except for the 0.8-mile side trip to the Wave Organ. Dogs must be leashed and their droppings picked up.

For more information: Contact the San Francisco Convention and Visitors Bureau or the GGNRA headquarters at Fort Mason.

Getting started: This walk begins at Fort Mason Center, located on San Francisco Bay just west of Fisherman's Wharf.

(1) For freeway exits into San Francisco from the East Bay or the San Francisco Peninsula, refer to "Meet San Francisco" earlier in this book. From the intersection of Market, Ninth, Hayes, and Larkin Streets near the Civic Center, veer left onto Hayes and go 3 blocks. Turn right onto Franklin Street and go almost 2 miles to Bay Street. Turn left onto Bay and follow the traffic as it turns right onto Laguna Street for 2 blocks and then left onto Beach Street for 1 block. At the stoplight at Beach, Buchanan Street, and Marina Boulevard, make a sharp right turn into the parking lot outside Fort Mason Center.

(2) From the Golden Gate Bridge, drive on U.S. Highway 101 South for about 1.5 miles and then veer left onto the Marina exit. Drive along Marina Boulevard for almost 2 miles to the stoplight at Marina Boulevard and Buchanan Street. Turn left at the light and then make an immediate right turn into the parking lot outside Fort Mason Center.

There is free parking—and designated wheelchair-accessible spaces—both within and just outside Fort Mason Center's gate, as well as along the Marina Green west of Fort Mason.

Public transportation: Bus 28 of the San Francisco Municipal Railway (Muni) stops at Fort Mason Center, and buses 22, 30, 42, 47, and 49 stop within 5 or 6 blocks of Fort Mason.

Marina Green

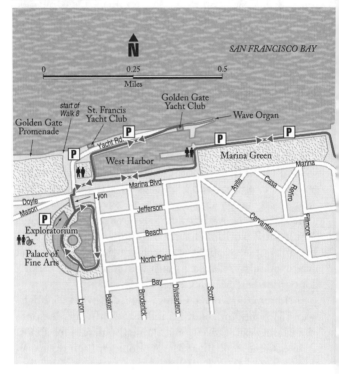

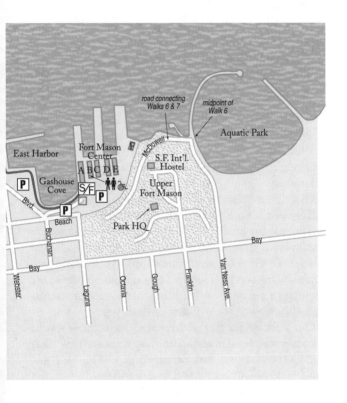

101

Buses 28 and 42 are wheelchair accessible. Contact Muni for information about schedules, fares, and accessibility.

Overview: Sailboats setting off for an afternoon jaunt around the bay, kites darting to and fro, joggers keeping a brisk pace, a sea breeze caressing your face: This bayside ramble makes the most of San Francisco's fabulous peninsula location. Bounded by water on three sides, the city—and its visitors—have ready access to some wonderful public spaces along the shore. The Marina Green is one of the most popular.

With its sweeping lawn, yacht harbors, and shoreline promenade, the Marina Green serves as a neighborhood park for the adjoining Marina District. You will see athletically inclined Marina residents—runners, skaters, cyclists, walkers—each time you visit the Green. Everyone is welcome to use the broad public pathways here—and the parcours stations set up along the way, for stretching those tight muscles. This is also a great place to bring your family, for a picnic or as a staging ground for an exhilarating visit to the Exploratorium, the kid-friendly science museum across Marina Boulevard at the Palace of Fine Arts.

Our walk begins at Fort Mason Center, one of several military installations in and around San Francisco now managed by the National Park Service as part of the magnificent Golden Gate National Recreation Area. In fact, the GGNRA's headquarters is here in Building 201, and you may want to stop in for information about this vast urban park, the largest of its kind in the world.

After passing by the Marina Green—with an optional side trip to a unique wave organ—the walk takes you to the Palace of Fine Arts, where you may opt to tour the Exploratorium's fascinating hands-on exhibits. You will finish by strolling back through the Green for one more taste of that salt air and the thrilling sight of all those sailboats swaying in their berths.

102

Note: Walk 7 can be combined with Walk 8—Golden Gate Promenade—for a 7-mile leg-stretching ramble along the bay. The two walks meet in the parking lot just to the west of the St. Francis Yacht Club. This spot marks the midpoint of Walk 7 and the start of Walk 8. To see exactly where in Walk 7 the start of Walk 8 occurs, see page 106.

The walk

►Start this walk on the south side of Fort Mason's Building A, just inside the wall that separates Fort Mason Center

of interest

Fort Mason Center

Fort Mason Center is a great "swords into plowshares" success. In use by the military for 200 years, the site was turned over to the National Park Service in 1972 and now serves as a lively community and cultural center.

Fort Mason Center is home to nearly 50 nonprofit groups, including museums, galleries, and theater groups. Among the organizations housed here are the Museo Italo-Americano, San Francisco Craft and Folk Art Museum, the San Francisco Museum of Modern Art Rental Gallery, Bay Area Theatersports, Magic Theater, and the Young Performers Theater. Fort Mason Center is also home to the Art Campus of the City College of San Francisco. The headquarters for the Golden Gate National Recreation Area is located at Upper Fort Mason, just to the southeast.

For the hungry, Fort Mason offers two excellent eating places: Cooks and Company in Building B, for takeout sandwiches, and the renowned Greens Restaurant in Building A overlooking Gashouse Cove, for the finest vegetarian meals anywhere.

from the yacht basin—called Gashouse Cove—and parking lot outside its gate.

➤Walk through the opening in Fort Mason's perimeter wall where it abuts Building A and descend the gentle ramp to the yacht harbor on Gashouse Cove.

➤Walk on the waterside sidewalk as it curves and turns around the perimeter of Gashouse Cove and East Harbor just beyond. These yacht basins, full of sparkling white and blue sailboats, are scenes of gentle motion and subtle sound. As the boats sway in the water, lines clink against masts, wooden docks creak, gulls call—and you may even hear a foghorn.

When the sidewalk nears Marina Green Drive, you will see the Marina Green up ahead. This long swath of green lawn is a popular weekend outing spot for San Franciscans—a great place for picnicking, kite flying, sunbathing, jogging, and walking.

➤Set out on the shoreline promenade.

There is another promenade that runs alongside Marina Boulevard on the opposite side of the green, but we much prefer the more scenic walkway along the water.

Just after passing a small building—the range house for the U.S. Naval Magnetic Silencing Range—in the middle of the open stretch of promenade, look out across the water. Directly opposite the range house is the jetty or spit of land that marks the endpoint of the side trip described on page 107. At low tide you can see a little beach and the stone Wave Organ at the end of the spit.

Designed by Peter Richards of the Exploratorium and constructed by stonemason and artist George Gonzales in 1986, the Wave Organ is made up of pipes that are "played" by the waves, producing music that varies with the tides and the size of the surf.

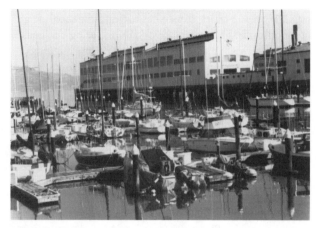

The sailboats of Gashouse Cove sway in their slips, with Fort Mason in the background.

Benches line the breakwater along the Marina Green's shoreline promenade. Take a moment to sit and join the gulls in contemplation of water, land, wind, and sky. In the middle of the bay lies Alcatraz Island; a bit farther out is the large mound of Angel Island; farthest away is the Marin County community of Tiburon, with fashionable houses sprinkled on its hillsides. The Golden Gate Bridge spans the waterway between San Francisco and Marin County to the north, and in the middle distance, a red tile roof marks the St. Francis Yacht Club.

➤Continue on the walkway as it turns left and walk past the eastern edge of West Harbor to Marina Boulevard.

Directly ahead, as you face the boulevard, you will see the distinctive architecture of the Marina District, a mix of Spanish tile roofs and pastel stucco homes and apartment buildings. Built on landfill that was deposited for the Panama Pacific International Exposition of 1915, the Marina was known as a quiet, somewhat boring residential neighborhood until the earthquake of 1989. During the quake, the landfill shook like jelly and brought a few buildings to their knees. Quickly rebuilt, the Marina is now one of the trendier neighborhoods for well-heeled young professionals.

When you reach Marina Boulevard, you will find yourself at an intersection with Scott Street and Cervantes Boulevard. There is a stoplight here. If you want to search out restaurants or shops on the return leg of this walk, make a note that both Cervantes and Scott lead to the busy neighborhood shopping district on Chestnut Street, 6 blocks to the south.

➤Turn right and walk along Marina Boulevard on the boulevard promenade. This noisy stretch of Marina Boulevard is one of the principal access routes to the Golden Gate Bridge.

Up ahead you will see the line of trees that marks the end of the westward progression of this walk. Look at the different types of boats in the West Harbor. Check to see whether there are any sailors rigging up for an afternoon race on the bay. Notice the trim joggers who make this their daily route. Ponder what it would be like to pull out of your driveway each morning into the traffic along Marina Boulevard.

➤At the end of the yacht harbor, turn right and walk on the broad asphalt path toward the bay and the St. Francis Yacht Club with its dignified stand of cypress. There are restrooms in the small building across the lawn.

➤Cross the parking lot on the west side of the St. Francis Yacht Club to reach the benches that overlook the bay.

For those who wish to combine Walk 7 with Walk 8, the Golden Gate Promenade, these bay-viewing benches mark the spot where the two walks meet. Walk 8 begins just to the left of the benches—as you face the bay—and leads off toward the Golden Gate Bridge.

Note: Those interested in taking a side trip to the Wave Organ should follow the directions below. The side trip is not wheelchair accessible and adds about a mile to the walk. If you prefer to bypass the side trip, turn to page 108 for the continuation of Walk 7.

Wave Organ Side Trip

➤With your back to the bay, retrace your steps across the parking lot and turn left to walk on the sidewalk between the yacht basin and the St. Francis Yacht Club.

This walk passes by the boat lift and the area where people rinse the salt water off their boats. You may need to step around gear and hoses on the walkway. Feel free to do so, and soak up the nautical local color.

➤Continue along the gravel walkway that hugs the yacht basin and leads toward a miniature stone lighthouse.

➤Walk across the end of the parking lot that lies to the east of the St. Francis Yacht Club, and walk to the left of the lighthouse which, with its crenellated tower, has a European feel.

➤Turn right and walk along the paved road that leads to the Golden Gate Yacht Club and the jetty beyond. A "Wave Organ" sign on the fence points down this road.

➤Pass Golden Gate Yacht Club and walk down the dirt road to the stone Wave Organ at the end of the jetty. Each time we visited, the organ was silent, but we loved the sights and sounds this far out on the bay.

Sit on a rock and listen to the waves slap against the breakwater, drink in the rich smell of ocean life, and watch the boats as they pass close by. Alcatraz Island lies not far away from your perch. There is an excellent view of Fort Mason and its yacht basin. Russian Hill is off to the right of Fort Mason. With water on three sides and exposed to the wind, you can easily imagine yourself out on the bay.

➤Retrace your steps to the St. Francis Yacht Club, the benches overlooking the bay at the edge of the parking lot, and the end of the Wave Organ Side Trip.

Note: Walk 7 continues at this point.

➤Leaving the benches behind, walk back to Marina Boulevard on the asphalt path along the edge of the yacht basin. Turn right onto the boulevard and walk 1 short block to the light and crosswalk.

➤Turn left and cross Marina Boulevard.

Take care in crossing. Despite the fact that there are stoplights at this intersection for the main roadway, drivers who continue straight ahead through the Presidio's Marina Gate on Mason Street sometimes do not stop for pedestrians.

➤Turn right and walk several yards to Lyon Street and the approach to the Palace of Fine Arts.

Those in wheelchairs, please note: The Palace of Fine Arts—and the Exploratorium that it houses—are wheelchair accessible, but there are no curb cuts allowing direct access to the building or grounds from the sidewalk along Lyon Street. To gain access, move into the parking lot and navigate carefully to the handicapped parking area in front of the large columns to the left of the Palace of Fine Arts' main building.

➤Turn left onto Lyon and walk 30 feet straight ahead on the sidewalk. When the sidewalk turns left into a private walkway, turn right, step over a grassy patch, and walk to the columns next to the designated handicapped parking.

The Palace of Fine Arts and the Exploratorium

In 1915, San Francisco sought to erase the memory of the 1906 earthquake and fire by throwing a world-class party. Known as the Panama Pacific International Exposition, this great fair officially celebrated the completion of the Panama Canal; but for San Franciscans, it also marked a return to normalcy and the rebuilding of their city.

Today, all that remains of the exposition is the Palace of Fine Arts, an extravagant Beaux Arts–style structure designed by famed Bay Area architect Bernard Maybeck. Originally built of lath and plaster, the palace—with its colonnades and rotunda—was resurrected in concrete in the mid-1960s.

The rotunda and its reflecting lake are wonderful to visit all on their own, but it is the exhibition hall next door that draws visitors by the millions. Here you will find the Palace of Fine Arts Theater and, more importantly, the Exploratorium, the science museum *Newsweek* has called one of the "great American amusement centers." Dedicated to making science accessible to everyone, the Exploratorium has been variously described as a "mad scientist's playpen" and the "wildest art show in town."

Prepare to be bombarded when you enter the Exploratorium. The folks who designed this hands-on science museum have done everything possible—and then some—to make sure that every visitor is engaged, bewildered, and delighted by each of the 650 interactive exhibits. Learn first-hand about the forces of weather, the structure of the human brain, and—in the Distorted Room and the Tactile Dome—the sometimes faulty testimony of your senses.

The Exploratorium Store, crowded with toys, books, and tools aimed at making science approachable, is a fascinating place in its own right—and a great place to stock up on gifts for the junior scientists in your life.

➤Walk beneath the columns, turn left, and stroll along the pathway as it curves toward the Palace of Fine Arts park and lagoon. A family of swans makes its home in the lagoon, and plenty of ducks and pigeons always hope for—and often receive—a handful of bread crumbs.

➤Circle this serene pond on the pathway, admire the antique charm of this flight of imagination from the first decades of the 20th century, and return to your starting point beneath the columns at the edge of the parking lot.

At this point, you may want to visit the Exploratorium, one of the Bay Area's premier attractions for kids—and anyone who loves science.

➤Retrace your steps to the corner of Lyon and Marina Boulevard and the nearby stoplight and crosswalk.

➤Cross Marina Boulevard at the stoplight, turn right, and retrace your steps past West Harbor, the Marina Green, East Harbor, and Gashouse Cove to Fort Mason and the end of this walk.

walk 8

Golden Gate Promenade

  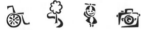

General location: Along the bay shoreline in north-central San Francisco, just east of the Golden Gate Bridge. Part of the Golden Gate National Recreation Area (GGNRA).

Special attractions: Historic fort; Golden Gate Bridge; beach, sand dunes, and tidal marsh; municipal fishing pier; picnicking; windsurfing.

Difficulty rating: Easy, flat, and entirely on sidewalks.

Distance: 3.5 miles.

Estimated time: 2 hours.

Services: Restrooms, picnic areas, visitor information center.

Restrictions: For wheelchair users: By mid-2000, the promenade will have been resurfaced with crushed stone rolled into place to create a firm surface with a natural appearance.

Golden Gate Promenade

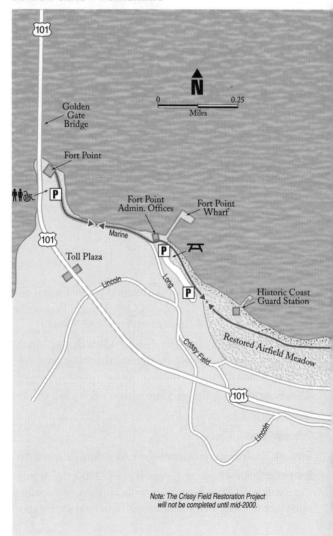

Note: The Crissy Field Restoration Project
will not be completed until mid-2000.

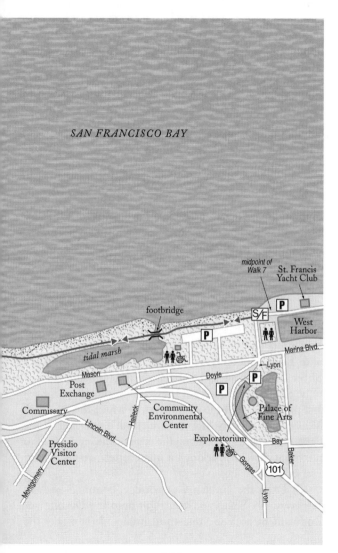

Until then, wheelchair users may encounter irregular surfaces, and the park service recommends they skip this walk until construction is completed. Dogs must either be leashed or under voice control, depending on where you are walking in the Golden Gate National Recreation Area. In some areas, pets are even prohibited entirely to protect sensitive resources. Dog droppings must be picked up. Contact the GGNRA headquarters at Fort Mason for pet regulations.

For more information: Contact the GGNRA headquarters at Fort Mason, the GGNRA Visitor Information Center at Fort Point, the GGNRA Visitor Information Center at the Presidio, or the San Francisco Convention and Visitors Bureau.

Getting started: This walk begins 1 block off Marina Boulevard, just west of the St. Francis Yacht Club, near the northeast corner of the Presidio of San Francisco.

(1) For freeway exits into San Francisco from the East Bay or the San Francisco Peninsula, refer to "Meet San Francisco" earlier in this book. From the intersection of Market, Ninth, Hayes, and Larkin Streets near the Civic Center, veer left onto Hayes, and go 3 blocks. Turn right onto Franklin Street and go almost 2 miles to Bay Street. Turn left onto Bay and follow the traffic as it curves onto Laguna Street, Beach Street, and then onto Marina Boulevard. Continue on Marina Boulevard for 8 blocks to the stoplight—just past the end of the boat harbor —where the Presidio's Mason Street meets Marina Boulevard. Turn right at the light and drive 1 block along the edge of the grassy field to reach the shoreline parking lot immediately west of the St. Francis Yacht Club.

(2) From the Golden Gate Bridge, continue on U.S. Highway 101 South and veer right onto the Downtown/Lombard turnoff. Go one-third mile and then take the

next possible right—a hairpin turn—onto Gorgas Avenue. Follow Gorgas about one-third mile through the Presidio. Turn right at Marshall Street and go 1 block, passing under US 101. Take the next right onto Mason Street. Drive about 3 blocks to the T junction just before the stoplight on Marina Boulevard. Turn left and drive along the edge of the grassy field for 1 block to reach the shoreline parking lot just west of the St. Francis Yacht Club.

Additional parking is available in the Golden Gate National Recreation Area parking lot between Mason Street and the shoreline, just west of where Mason meets Marina Boulevard.

Public transportation: Bus 30 of the San Francisco Municipal Railway (Muni) stops at the corner of Broderick and Jefferson streets, 4 blocks from the start of this walk. Bus 30 is not wheelchair accessible. Contact Muni for information about schedules and fares.

Overview: Yet another pleasurable saunter along the shore of San Francisco Bay, this walk takes you down a stretch of beach that was once a vast dune field edged by salt marshes and lagoons. Until recently a landing strip and military work yard, this area is now—in an astonishing feat of environmental restoration—being returned to a condition that closely resembles its original state. Known as the Crissy Field Restoration Project, this effort involves the National Park Service's Golden Gate National Recreation Area (GGNRA); the GGNRA's nonprofit support partner, the Golden Gate National Parks Association; and several private foundations.

Used for many years as a military airfield, Crissy Field was built in the 1920s when flying was still young. Constructed in peacetime and predating the U.S. Air Force, the field housed the air squadron based at the Presidio, which used it for fire patrols and aerial photography flights.

In the restoration process, the Army has thoroughly cleared the 100-acre Crissy Field area of hazardous substances. With this cleanup completed, the Golden Gate National Parks Association is now engaged in restoring the wild, open character of this shoreline. This means that the beaches are being cleaned and expanded, the promenade widened and given a new surface, a tidal marsh extending over 20 acres thoroughly restored to its natural state, the dunes replanted with native species, and the airfield pavement removed and replaced with a grassy meadow.

We have written this walk based on the Golden Gate National Parks Association's final design for the shoreline park. If you visit before mid-2000, you may encounter some temporary detours, and the planned facilities and interpretive signage may not yet be complete. However, do not hesitate to embark on this walk. Detours or not, this stretch of bayshore is still a wonderful place to amble. And as the association notes in a recent press release, the restoration has been designed "to have as little impact as possible on regular and seasonal users of the space."

Besides taking you along this beautifully restored shoreline, the Golden Gate Promenade leads you past a historic Coast Guard station, out onto a public fishing pier, and to Fort Point, the mid-19th-century brick fortification just beneath the southern end of the Golden Gate Bridge.

Note: Walk 8 can be combined with Walk 7—Marina Green—for a 7-mile leg-stretching ramble along the bay. The two walks meet in the parking lot just to the west of the St. Francis Yacht Club. This spot marks the start of Walk 8 and the midpoint of Walk 7. To see exactly where in Walk 7 the start of Walk 8 occurs, see page 106.

The walk

➤Start the walk at the benches overlooking the bay at the edge of the parking lot on the west side of the St. Francis Yacht Club.

➤Face the bay and then walk left onto the promenade which heads off along the water toward the Golden Gate Bridge. Immediately as you step onto the promenade, you enter another world—a world of sand dunes, salt air, wind, and waves.

➤Continue on the promenade as it passes restored sand dunes and the beach that lies beyond.

This stretch of beach and bay is one of the most popular windsurfing areas in the world. Stiff breezes and strong bay currents make it a challenging spot—most definitely not one for the novice. Experienced windsurfers may make it look easy to skim across the water like a waterbug going 25 to 30 knots—or about 30 to 35 miles per hour. However, if you see someone less experienced struggling to stay upright, you will begin to appreciate the level of strength and skill it takes to have fun on these waters.

➤Cross the small footbridge that marks the opening of the tidal marsh onto the bay.

This tidal marsh is new, yet old. Originally marshland, this area was later filled in and paved to serve as part of the airfield at Crissy Field. Look for birds and animals that have discovered this rich natural habitat since its recent restoration.

➤Just beyond the bridge is one of several paths that lead through the sand dunes to the beach.

To preserve this carefully nurtured habitat, stay on the paths between planted areas as you move between the promenade and the beach. If you like, wander down a dune path and walk on the beach for a while. You will find other paths leading back to the promenade at various points along the beach.

Despite the proximity of the airfield and the public's use of this area as an informal park for many years, these dunes have always maintained a small community of native plants. The National Park Service has recently given nature a boost, planting more than 55,000 native plants on these dunes and in the marsh. Prominent among the native species on the dunes is *Elymus mollis,* a thick green grass hardy enough to thrive in the strong winds and chill fogs of this site.

➤Continue on the promenade past the tidal marsh and then past a large grassy meadow that until recently was covered with the tarmac of Crissy Field.

➤At the end of the meadow, pass the historic Coast Guard station. The station's residence dates from 1890 and the boathouse from 1919. The Gulf of the Farallones National Marine Sanctuary has recently opened a visitor center at the station.

➤Continue on the promenade as it draws close to the water's edge and heads toward Fort Point Wharf, built in 1908 and used today as a public fishing pier.

Head out on the pier to get a closer look at how shore-line fishing is done on the San Francisco Bay. The uneven surface of the pier becomes less hospitable to wheelchairs the farther out you go.

➤Follow the promenade as it passes around the Fort Point Administrative Offices and joins Marine Drive on its way to the Civil War–era Fort Point.

➤Walk along the broad shoulder of Marine Drive toward Fort Point, the austere-looking brick building at the foot of the Golden Gate Bridge. Waves crash against the breakwater just to your right, and occasionally you will see surfers nearby.

of interest

Fort Point

There is something irresistible, even haunting, about an old fortification, and Fort Point is no exception. Here, just beneath the southern end of the Golden Gate Bridge, this massive structure made of brick and stone guards the entrance—the Golden Gate—to San Francisco Bay.

Spanish troops first built a fort, El Castillo de San Joaquin, here in 1793. When Mexico claimed its independence from Spain in 1821, the Mexican army took over the adobe fort. In 1848, following the Mexican War, the United States acquired California, and soon an American gun battery replaced the old Spanish fortifications.

The structure we visit today was built between 1853 and 1861. Designed to withstand bombardments by the most powerful cannon of the time, Fort Point boasts walls that are 5 to 7 feet thick. Ninety gun rooms, called casemates, once held as many as 102 cannon and a few mortars and gave this great fort plenty of firepower.

Changes in technology—the emergence of ironclad gunships, rifled guns, and giant smoothbore cannon—soon rendered Fort Point vulnerable, and by the end of the Civil War, it had become obsolete. Other batteries at Fort Mason, on Angel and Alcatraz Islands, along the cliffs of the Presidio, and in the Marin Headlands took over the defense of San Francisco and its bay.

Today Fort Point, which never saw action, stands as a monument to a vanished kind of warfare and to the artillery- and infantrymen who made certain that San Francisco was well defended.

To learn more about this landmark, you can take a tour led by a ranger or park volunteer, follow a self-guided tour, or rent a tour on tape. For more information about tours, ask a ranger or inquire at the Golden Gate National Parks Association store on the fort's first floor.

➤Once you reach Fort Point, go around to the right of the building for an intimate view of the colossal bridge from directly underneath its great span. Look out over the water to get a sense of the power of the currents that pass through the Golden Gate. Look beyond the bridge to glimpse the wide and majestic Pacific Ocean.

➤Return to the entrance of Fort Point, and walk into the main courtyard to see this odd-shaped structure—it has five sides—from the interior. Stairs lead to exhibits on the upper floors and then to the rooftop level. There is no elevator access. The roof offers dramatic views of the bridge, the bay, the city, and the ocean. It is often very windy up here and the drop is fairly unprotected, so hold onto your hat and your kids.

➤Exit Fort Point and return along the roadway to the shoreline promenade. Retrace your steps past the Coast Guard station, the grassy meadow, and the tidal marsh.

➤Continue on the shoreline promenade back to the parking lot near the St. Francis Yacht Club and the end of this walk.

walk 9

Golden Gate Bridge and Baker Beach

   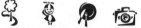

General location: In northwestern San Francisco, just south of Golden Gate Bridge. Part of the Golden Gate National Recreation Area (GGNRA).

Special attractions: Golden Gate Bridge; beach; clifftop views of San Francisco, ocean, and bay; military landmarks.

Difficulty rating: Moderate, with some steep uphill. The trail surface is frequently uneven.

Distance: 3 miles.

Estimated time: 1.5 hours.

Services: Parking, restrooms, snack bar.

Restrictions: Not wheelchair accessible. Be careful on cliffs and at the beach. This part of the coast is known for its

Golden Gate Bridge and Baker Beach

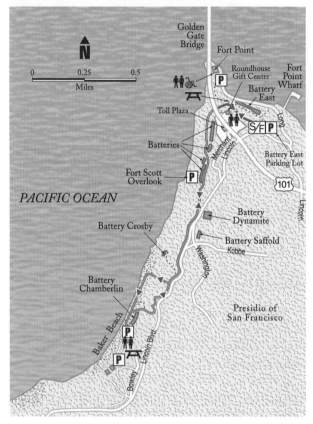

strong riptides, and Baker Beach is posted "Hazardous Surf—Swim at Your Own Risk." Each year the National Park Service rescues numerous people—and dogs—who fall off cliffs or get swept away by heavy surf or riptides. Dogs must either be leashed or under voice control, depending on where you are walking in the Golden Gate National Recreation Area. In some areas, pets are even prohibited entirely to protect sensitive resources. Dog droppings must be picked up. Contact the GGNRA headquarters at Fort Mason for pet regulations.

For more information: Contact GGNRA headquarters at Fort Mason or the Presidio Visitor Information Center.

Getting started: This walk begins at the Battery East parking lot located near the Golden Gate Bridge toll plaza in the Presidio of San Francisco.

(1) For directions into San Francisco from the East Bay or the San Francisco Peninsula, refer to "Meet San Francisco" earlier in this book. From the intersection of Market, Ninth, Hayes, and Larkin Streets, veer left onto Hayes and go 3 blocks. Turn right onto Franklin Street and go about 1.75 miles to Lombard Street. Turn left onto Lombard and go 11 blocks to Broderick Street, ending up in the left-hand lane. Just after Broderick, as the traffic curves to the right, remain on Lombard and follow the sign at the stoplight to the Presidio. Continue 1.5 blocks on Lombard and enter the Presidio through the Lombard Gate. Turn right onto Presidio Boulevard at the first stop sign. Continue straight through several stop signs. You are now on Lincoln Boulevard. As you pass the foot of the Presidio's main parade ground, follow signs for the Golden Gate Bridge. At the next stop, turn right onto Sheridan Avenue. You will pass the San Francisco National Cemetery, after which you rejoin Lincoln. Continue on Lincoln for about 1 mile—past the

turnoff to Fort Point at Long Avenue—and then turn right into the Battery East parking lot.

Note: Interstate 280 North offers an alternate and more direct route from the San Francisco Peninsula. After passing through Daly City on I-280 North, take the Golden Gate Bridge/19th Avenue exit and drive on California Highway 1 North—along Junipero Serra Boulevard, 19th Avenue, and Park Presidio Boulevard—for about 5 miles. One block after crossing Geary Street, turn right onto Clement Street and then take an immediate right onto Funston Avenue. Go 1 block, turn right onto Geary, and cross Park Presidio. Continue on Geary for 11 blocks to 25th Avenue. Turn right onto 25th and go 4 blocks to Lincoln Boulevard. Turn right onto Lincoln and go about 1.75 miles. Just after passing under an overpass for U.S. Highway 101, turn left into the Battery East parking lot.

(2) From the Golden Gate Bridge, pass through the far right toll booth and take an immediate right onto the 25th Avenue exit. Turn left at the first stop sign onto Lincoln Boulevard, drive one-quarter mile, and turn left into the Battery East parking lot.

Public transportation: San Francisco Municipal Railway (Muni) buses 28 and 29 stop in the visitor parking lot at the south end of Golden Gate Bridge near the Roundhouse Gift Center and Bridge Cafe. Contact Muni for information about schedules, fares, and accessibility. To join the walk route, go past the statue of Joseph Strauss, bridge engineer, turn right at the Men of Vision monument, and walk a short distance to an intersection with a wide asphalt trail. Turn left onto this asphalt trail to begin the walk soon after its start at the Battery East parking lot.

Overview: Combining a gorgeous natural setting with unusual views of the Golden Gate Bridge and glimpses of military history, this walk is among our San Francisco favorites. Certainly, the most dramatic attraction here is the nearly 2-mile-long Art Deco bridge, one of the city's most identifiable landmarks. Having turned 50 in 1987, the Golden Gate Bridge is a tangible symbol of the vitality, elegance, and strength of the city by the bay.

The walk begins just above Fort Point, a massive brick structure erected between 1853 and 1861 to guard San Francisco from attack by enemy warships. Early in the walk, you will pass by the ruins of gun emplacements built in the early 20th century. Also intended to defend the narrow entrance to San Francisco Bay, these mysterious and lonely-looking batteries offer additional testimony to San Francisco's key role as a port and commercial center.

For walkers, however, it is this trail's natural beauty that will most appeal. As you walk along the oceanside cliffs, past grassy fields and through groves of eucalyptus and cypress, you will experience firsthand the wild freedom of the Pacific coast—and you will come to understand its fragility. These cliffs are part of the Presidio of San Francisco, the former military reservation now managed by the National Park Service. For another amble through the Presidio, see Walk 16. The park service is doing everything possible to preserve the threatened and endangered native plants and animals that reside on these cliffs and beaches. Please aid in these preservation efforts by staying on the main trail.

Baker Beach—the midpoint of this walk—offers a quintessential San Francisco beach experience. As you walk the sandy beach, enjoy the pungent ocean air; watch the antics of children, dogs, and fisherfolk; and delight in the crash of waves and the sight of shorebirds skittering at water's edge.

The walk

➤Start this walk on the broad asphalt trail near the entrance to the Battery East parking lot in the Presidio of San Francisco. Walk on the trail away from the parking lot and toward Golden Gate Bridge.

On your right, you will pass the series of concrete gun emplacements known as Battery East.

On your left, you will soon pass two turnoffs that lead to the Roundhouse Gift Center and Bridge Cafe, public restrooms, and the beginning of the pedestrian walkway across the Golden Gate Bridge.

Note: Those taking public transportation to the Roundhouse Gift Center will join the trail here. See "Public transportation" above.

Notice the exotic plantings along this section of the path, especially the fantastically shaped pride of Madeira, with its blossoms on tall spikes.

➤Continue on the asphalt path and pass beneath the Golden Gate Bridge. Here you will hear the steady rumble of bridge traffic heading to and from Marin County.

➤Shortly after passing under the bridge, turn right off the paved path and onto the dirt path marked "Coastal Trail."

Cyclists, take note: The paved path you have just departed soon makes a hairpin curve to the left, and a sign announces "Bicyclists Only—No Pedestrians Beyond This Point." This excellent paved path allows cyclists to cross the Golden Gate Bridge on its western side, during those hours when bicycle traffic is restricted to this side—Monday through Friday, 3:30 P.M. to 9 P.M., and Saturday, Sunday, and holidays, 5 A.M. to 9 P.M.

➤Continue straight ahead on the dirt path, and as you come into the open, you suddenly will have gorgeous views of the

of interest

Golden Gate Bridge

Perhaps the most photogenic—and photographed—bridge in the world, the Golden Gate Bridge is a vivid and compelling emblem. Whenever we encounter its image, we think instantly of San Francisco.

Built by engineer Joseph Strauss and designed by architect Irving Morrow, the bridge took more than four years to build, from 1933 to 1937, and cost $35 million. Its span of 6,450 feet was the longest in the world at the time of its completion, and the cable that keeps it suspended would stretch 80,000 miles, or three times around the earth, were it to come unspun.

This feat of engineering and artistry carries more than 100,000 vehicles to and from the city each day. Pedestrians and bicyclists often crowd the walkway on the bridge's east side, while the sidewalk on the west side is reserved for bicyclists only during limited hours. Many cyclists then take their mountain bikes into the Marin Headlands (see Walk 17). If you want to walk across the bridge—about 1.7 miles each way—set out from the Roundhouse Gift Center near the beginning of this walk. You can also take a Golden Gate Transit bus across the bridge in either direction. The northbound bus pad is located near the bridge toll plaza. Take a Sausalito-bound bus. The southbound bus pad is one-quarter mile beyond the northern end of the bridge, along the road leading to Sausalito.

Golden Gate Bridge behind you and, off to your right and ahead, the staggeringly beautiful cliffs of the Pacific Coast. You will find the back side of another set of concrete gun emplacements—Battery Cranston—off to your left. Directly across the water lie the Marin Headlands. The headlands, also part of the Golden Gate National Recreation Area, are explored in Walks 17 and 18.

Please resist the temptation to depart the main trail for the inviting social (non-official) trails that lead to the edge of the cliffs. While the main trail is safe, some of the informal overlooks may not be—coastal cliffs are unstable and the surf is treacherous.

►Follow the trail up a wooden staircase. You will pass the first of several native plant restoration sites along this walk. This site, part of the Serpentine Bluff Restoration Project, is habitat to two rare plant species, coast rock cress and San Francisco gum plant. Serpentine habitats, underlain by serpentinite, the state mineral of California, once stretched in a band across the San Francisco Peninsula. Development has wiped out most of these habitats. The only remnants survive on a few acres in the Presidio, here and on Inspiration Point, which is included in Walk 16.

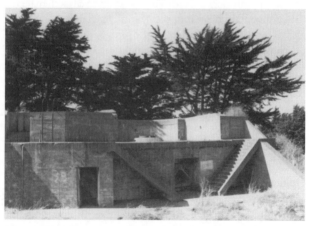

The gun batteries along the Presidio's clifftops are quiet ruins today.

of interest

Coastal Gun Emplacements

Since Europeans first set foot in the Bay Area, they have sought to defend this great natural harbor from ocean-going enemies. As early as 1776, Spanish troops set up fortifications bristling with cannon where Forts Point and Mason stand today.

During the Mexican War, the U.S. Army began to plan its own forts here, at Fort Point, at Lime Point—in the Marin Headlands—and on Alcatraz Island. By the Civil War, changes in technology had made massive forts like Fort Point obsolete, and less expensive and substantial batteries defended the bay from Fort Mason and Angel Island.

Between the late 19th century and World War II, the military installed a series of ever more powerful and accurate guns along the cliffs of the Presidio. These are the batteries you see today as you walk from the Golden Gate Bridge to Baker Beach.

As you pass these forlorn ruins—Batteries East, Boutelle, Godfrey, Dynamite, Crosby, and Chamberlin—imagine the days when troops manned these gun emplacements, waiting in vain for the attack that never came.

➤After you pass Battery Boutelle and Battery Godfrey on your right, watch for the park service sign for the Coastal Trail. Turn right just beyond the sign and continue on the narrow dirt trail.

➤Soon the trail meets an access road that leads to a parking lot and Fort Scott Overlook. Cross the road to the small "hiker" sign, and continue on the trail as it veers to the left and passes through a grove of Monterey pine.

➤Continue on the trail as it turns right and runs alongside Lincoln Boulevard for one-third mile. As you join Lincoln Boulevard, try to spot the vegetation-covered gun emplacement—Battery Dynamite—hidden in the hillside across the roadway.

➤Pass the turnoff to Battery Crosby and then turn right onto the trail marked "Beach Access."

➤Follow the trail as it steeply descends a tall and broad sand dune. The plants alongside the trail are important to dune stabilization and to wildlife. They can be easily destroyed by trampling; please stay on the trail.

At the top of this immense and majestic dune, take a moment, breathe deep, and drink it all in: the undulating ocean, the far-off horizon, Baker Beach below, Golden Gate Bridge, and the rough cliffs of the Marin Headlands across the water. Off to your left, just beyond the beach, you will see the posh residential district of Seacliff. Beyond Seacliff lies Lands End, the tree-clad western tip of the San Francisco Peninsula explored in Walk 11.

➤At the bottom of the dune, walk left along the beach past two trails that lead back up the hillside. You can use either of these two trails for your return to Lincoln Boulevard.

Baker Beach has a friendly, relaxed feeling, like a neighborhood park. Even on a cloudy, windy day, the beach is busy. Families relax on the sand, and fisherfolk stick their long surf-casting poles in the sand, catching perch, smelt, striped bass, and skate.

➤A third path leading away from the beach goes to the beach parking lot and to Battery Chamberlin.

Battery Chamberlin, yet another coastal fortification, is known for its 50-ton "disappearing" gun, the last operational gun of its kind. After being fired, the giant cannon drops below the battery wall to allow its crew to reload in safety from enemy fire. On the first weekend of each month, a park ranger, assisted by volunteers in period uniform, demonstrates how the disappearing gun operates. Contact the GGNRA headquarters at Fort Mason for dates and times.

➤For your return trip, ascend either of the two paths mentioned earlier that lie between the parking lot and the beach access trail that you descended. These two trails meet at an old roadbed that winds up through a grove of Monterey pine to Lincoln Boulevard.

➤When you reach Lincoln Boulevard, turn left onto the roadside path and retrace your steps to the Battery East parking lot and the end of this walk. From this direction, you will have one more chance to appreciate the land- and seascapes of this spectacular stretch of Pacific coast.

Ocean Beach and Lands End

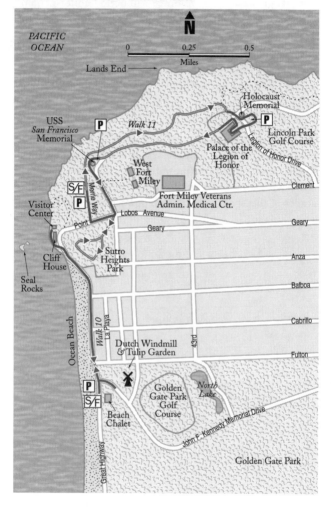

walk 10

Ocean Beach

General location: In northwestern San Francisco, on the western edge of Golden Gate Park, along the Pacific Ocean. Includes part of the Golden Gate National Recreation Area (GGNRA).

Special attractions: Beach walking, sea lion and shorebird viewing, amusement park novelties, historic architecture, murals, formal garden.

Difficulty rating: Easy.

Distance: 1.25 miles.

Estimated time: 45 minutes.

Services: Parking, restaurants, restrooms, visitor information centers.

Restrictions: Wheelchair accessible only along Ocean Beach Esplanade. The hill up to the Cliff House is rather steep, but still accessible for many wheelchair strollers. Dogs must be leashed and their droppings picked up. On Ocean Beach, dogs are allowed under voice control from Stairwell 1 south to Stairwell 21; beyond Stairwell 21, dogs must be leashed to protect the endangered western snowy plover. Be careful on cliffs and at the beach. Each year, the park service rescues numerous people—and dogs—who fall off cliffs or get swept away by heavy surf or riptides.

For more information: Contact the Golden Gate National Recreation Area (GGNRA) Visitor Information Center at the Cliff House or the Golden Gate Park Visitor Information Center at the Beach Chalet.

Getting started: This walk starts at the entrance to the historic Beach Chalet, on the Great Highway at the western edge of Golden Gate Park.

(1) For freeway exits into San Francisco from the East Bay or the San Francisco Peninsula, refer to "Meet San Francisco" earlier in this book. From the intersection of Market, Ninth, Hayes, and Larkin Streets near the Civic Center, veer left onto Hayes and go 3 blocks. Turn right onto Franklin Street and go 9 blocks. Turn left onto Geary Boulevard and drive approximately 5 miles to the Pacific Ocean. In the last half mile, veer right with the traffic onto Point Lobos Avenue. Once at ocean level, continue on the Great Highway for about one-half mile to the Beach Chalet, 1.5 blocks beyond Fulton Street.

Interstate 280 North offers an alternate and more direct route from the San Francisco Peninsula. After passing through Daly City on I-280 North, take the Golden Gate Bridge/19th Avenue exit and drive on California Highway 1 North—along Junipero Serra Boulevard, 19th Avenue, and Park Presidio Boulevard—for about 4 miles to Irving Street. Turn right onto Irving and go 1 block. Turn left onto 18th

Avenue and go 1 block. Turn left onto Lincoln Way and drive 2 miles to the Pacific Ocean. Turn right onto the Great Highway and drive about one-half mile to the Beach Chalet.

(2) From the Golden Gate Bridge: Pass through the far right toll booth and take an immediate right onto the 25th Avenue exit. At the first stop sign, turn right onto Lincoln Boulevard and drive on Lincoln for about 1.5 miles. Just after Lincoln emerges from the Presidio, turn left onto 25th Avenue and go 4 blocks. Turn right onto Geary Boulevard and drive approximately 1.5 miles to the Pacific Ocean. In the last half mile, veer right with the traffic onto Point Lobos Avenue. Once at ocean level, continue on the Great Highway for about one-half mile to the Beach Chalet, 1.5 blocks beyond Fulton Street.

Park directly in front of the Beach Chalet or in the ample lot between the Great Highway and the ocean.

Public transportation: Buses 5, 31, and 38 (Ocean Beach route) of the San Francisco Municipal Railway (Muni) run from downtown to the corner of LaPlaya and Cabrillo Streets, roughly 2 blocks north of the Beach Chalet. Contact Muni for information about schedules, fares, and accessibility.

Overview: Kids will love this walk. So will adults who cannot resist beaches, the Pacific Ocean, and San Francisco's fabled Cliff House, with its intriguing Camera Obscura and museum of mechanical wonders, the Musée Mecanique.

You begin your stroll—this is definitely not a vigorous hike—at the recently renovated Beach Chalet across from Ocean Beach. This walk then takes you briefly into Golden Gate Park, for a visit to a Dutch windmill and tulip garden, and then leads you across the Great Highway to one of San Francisco's finest public beaches.

Ocean Beach, a sandy expanse gently inclining toward the Pacific Ocean, invites all and sundry to escape the noise and density of the city. Families set up beach umbrellas and lay out picnics; dogs walk their owners near water's edge; gulls convene in the sand; kids guide their kites high above; and bicyclists and in-line skaters gracefully wheel along the esplanade.

If you can tear yourself away from the beach's pleasures, head up the esplanade to one of San Francisco's most romantic attractions. The Cliff House, despite its current seedy charm, recalls an elegant seaside resort of the early 20th century. A meal in its second-story restaurant, high above the Pacific, is always memorable. Targeted for massive remodeling, the Cliff House will soon be irresistible—restored to its original elegance and size, with the Musée Mecanique and Camera Obscura relocated nearby and the surroundings generally spiffed up.

Kids of all ages will thrill to the "World Famous" Musée Mecanique, home to hundreds of antique musical and mechanical toys and games: Laughing Sal, whose infectious and terrifying laughter will send shivers up your spine; a Ferris wheel built by inmates in San Quentin Prison; "The Unbelievable Mechanical Farm"; and player pianos, mechanical belly dancers, and old-time gambling devices, to name just a few. Founded by Edward Galland Zelinsky—"collector, restorer, and preserver of fascinating antique automata"—Musée Mecanique is crowded and noisy and absolutely enchanting.

On the oceanside plaza surrounding the Cliff House, shed the carnival atmosphere of the mechanical museum and allow yourself to be mesmerized by the sound and sight of the rolling breakers. When you have had your fill, stroll down the beach one last time before returning to the city's clamor.

Note: For a longer stroll of an additional 3 miles, this walk may be combined with Walk 11, Lands End. One long block along Point Lobos Avenue—between the Cliff House, the midpoint of Walk 10, and Merrie Way, the start of Walk 11—links one walk to the other. See page 140 to pinpoint where this link occurs in Walk 10.

The walk

➤Start at the entrance to the Beach Chalet, located on the Great Highway near the corner of Fulton Street.

The Beach Chalet was built in 1925 to house a restaurant and changing rooms for Ocean Beach bathers. Designed by architect Willis Polk in the Spanish Colonial style, the chalet was decorated in the late 1930s by muralist Lucien Labaudt. Labaudt's lively San Francisco scenes—commissioned by the Works Progress Administration—survive today; the building, renovated in 1996, is once again home to a restaurant—with microbrewery—on its upper floor. The Golden Gate Park Visitor Information Center is on the ground floor.

➤Enter the Beach Chalet to visit the visitor center and to view Labaudt's murals.

➤Exit the Beach Chalet by its front door, turn right, and walk north about 500 feet along the Great Highway to John F. Kennedy Drive.

➤Cross John F. Kennedy Drive, turn right, and walk up the sidewalk to the Dutch Windmill.

The windmill was built in 1903 to pump water from freshwater wells to irrigate Golden Gate Park and, in the words of the Park Commission, to "lend to the landscape a picturesque feature." A second windmill, the Murphy Windmill, was built to the south, but by 1913 wind power was replaced by the new electrical age and its motorized pumps. The Dutch Windmill was restored in 1981; the Murphy Windmill is still in disrepair.

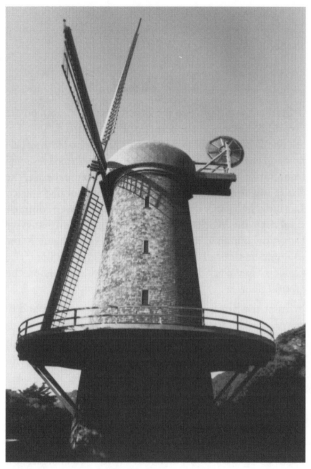

The Dutch Windmill once pumped water to irrigate Golden Gate Park.

➤Walk into the Queen Wilhelmina Tulip Garden adjacent to the windmill.

Whatever the season and even on the foggiest San Francisco morning, this garden sparkles with bright colors laid out in orderly patterns. In early spring (February or March), you will find a dazzling display of tulips, as many as 10,000 of them. A host of other flowering plants bloom here during the remainder of the year.

➤Return to the Great Highway, turn right, and walk a partial block to Fulton Street. Cross the Great Highway with the light at Fulton.

➤Turn right and walk along the esplanade toward the Cliff House, the building perched on the hill above the ocean. For those wishing to walk at the water's edge, we recommend that you descend to Ocean Beach at one of the many stairways cut into the concrete retaining wall along the esplanade. Although you may see people in the water, Ocean Beach is known for its riptides, and swimming can be extremely dangerous. The beach itself is not wheelchair accessible.

➤Walk along the esplanade as it climbs toward the Cliff House. Just before reaching the Cliff House, turn left off the main sidewalk and walk onto the walkway that circles behind the building.

Stop and look over the wall at dizzying views of breakers hitting the rocks below. Look back at the great stretch of Ocean Beach. From this vantage point, you can see both windmills in Golden Gate Park. Until 1972, the area just this side of the Beach Chalet, where a modern apartment complex now stands, was the site of Playland at the Beach, a well-known amusement park.

➤Continue on the walkway to the oceanside plaza behind the Cliff House.

Look out over the ocean, and listen for the barking of the California sea lions that congregate on Seal Rocks just offshore. Watch the surfers testing the waves at Ocean Beach. You may also see a fishing boat heading out to sea or a freighter on the horizon. Below the cliffs visible from the plaza's north end, you will spot the ruins of the historic Sutro Baths.

Located on the ocean side of the plaza is the giant Camera Obscura and Holograph Gallery, a remnant of Playland at the Beach. Claimed to be the world's biggest camera, the rotating San Francisco Camera Obscura captures haunting images of its surroundings—the plaza, the Seal Rocks, sunsets—on a large parabolic screen. Along the Cliff House's rear wall is the entrance to the Musée Mecanique.

➤Opposite the entrance to the Musée Mecanique you will find one of the Golden Gate National Recreation Area's well-stocked visitor information centers. There are wheelchair-accessible restrooms near the entrance to the visitor center.

➤Retrace your steps across the oceanside plaza and rejoin the esplanade, which passes in front of the Cliff House. You may want to step inside the Cliff House for a drink, a meal, or a visit to the gift shop.

For those who wish to combine Walk 10 with Walk 11, Lands End, continue uphill on Point Lobos Avenue another long block to the Merrie Way parking lot. Walk 11 starts at the trailhead at the far end of the parking lot and ends at the entrance to this parking lot.

➤Walk down the esplanade to Ocean Beach. When you have finished with any last-minute beachcombing, return to the start of your walk at the Beach Chalet.

walk 11

Lands End

(See map on page 132)

General location: In northwestern San Francisco, along the Pacific Ocean, just north of Ocean Beach and the Cliff House. Includes part of the Golden Gate National Recreation Area (GGNRA).

Special attractions: Natural landscapes, ocean and city views, museum, monuments, historic park.

Difficulty rating: Moderate, on dirt paths.

Distance: 3 miles.

Estimated time: 1.5 hours.

Services: Restaurants, restrooms, visitor information center.

Restrictions: Not wheelchair accessible. Be careful on cliffs and at the beach. Each year, the National Park Service rescues numerous people—and dogs—who fall off cliffs or get swept away by heavy surf or riptides. Dogs must either be leashed or under voice control, depending on where you are walking in the Golden Gate National Recreation Area. In some areas, pets are even prohibited entirely to protect sensitive resources. Dog droppings must be picked up. Contact the GGNRA headquarters at Fort Mason for a listing of pet regulations.

For more information: Contact the GGNRA headquarters office at Fort Mason; the GGNRA Visitor Information Center at the Cliff House; or the California Palace of the Legion of Honor.

Getting started: This walk begins at the parking lot on Merrie Way, off Point Lobos Avenue on the Pacific Ocean just above the Cliff House.

(1) For freeway exits into San Francisco from the East Bay or the San Francisco Peninsula, refer to "Meet San Francisco" earlier in this book. From the intersection of Market, Ninth, Hayes, and Larkin Streets near the Civic Center, veer left onto Hayes and go 3 blocks. Turn right onto Franklin Street and go 9 blocks. Turn left onto Geary Boulevard and drive approximately 5 miles to the Pacific Ocean. In the last half mile, veer right with the traffic onto Point Lobos Avenue. Continue on Point Lobos for three-quarters of a mile, turn right on Merrie Way, and park in the lot.

Interstate 280 North offers an alternate and more direct route from the San Francisco Peninsula. After passing through Daly City on I-280 North, take the Golden Gate Bridge/19th Avenue exit and drive on California Highway 1 North—along Junipero Serra Boulevard, 19th Avenue, and Park Presidio Boulevard—for about 4 miles to Irving Street. Turn right onto Irving and go 1 block. Turn left onto 18th Avenue and go 1 block. Turn left onto Lincoln Way and drive 2 miles to the Pacific Ocean. Turn right onto the Great Highway and drive about 1 mile. Follow the traffic north onto Point Lobos Avenue as it winds up past the Cliff House. About 1 block past the Cliff House, turn left onto Merrie Way and park in the lot.

(2) From the Golden Gate Bridge: Pass through the far right toll booth and take an immediate right onto the 25th Avenue exit. Turn right at the first stop sign onto Lincoln Boulevard. Drive on Lincoln for about 1.5 miles. Turn left onto 25th Avenue just after Lincoln emerges from the Presidio, and go 4 blocks. Turn right onto Geary Boulevard and drive approximately 5 miles to the Pacific Ocean. In the last half mile, veer right with the traffic onto Point Lobos Avenue. Continue on Point Lobos for three-quarters of a mile, turn right onto Merrie Way, and park in the lot.

Public transportation: Buses 5, 31, and 38 (Ocean Beach route) of the San Francisco Municipal Railway (Muni) run from downtown to the corner of LaPlaya and Cabrillo Streets, roughly 4 blocks below the Cliff House. Transfer to the northbound bus 18, and then debark 5 blocks later across from the Merrie Way parking lot. Contact Muni for information about schedules, fares, and accessibility.

Overview: Besides a good, but not exhausting workout, this walk offers cliffside views of the Pacific, a magnificent museum, and one of San Francisco's best-kept secrets—magical Sutro Heights Park. It should also allay any doubts you might harbor about the importance of the Golden Gate National Recreation Area to San Francisco's quality of life. Starting just uphill from the fabled Cliff House and the ruins of Sutro Baths, the walk leads you along the Coastal Trail. This clearly defined pathway provides both broad vistas and intimate glimpses of passing freighters, the remnants of shipwrecks, and the ever-enticing ocean. Because the cliffsides can be unstable, stay on the trail at all times and keep a close eye on the children in your party.

Midway through the walk, you will emerge from the coastal forest into Lincoln Park, where golf carts and caddies wend their way across groomed greens. Also in view will be the California Palace of the Legion of Honor, one of San Francisco's fine city museums. Upon leaving the Palace, you will reenter the forest and follow a trail higher up the hillside than the Coastal Trail, but just as beautiful. There you will encounter a moving memorial to the World War II heroics of the USS *San Francisco*.

Near the walk's end, you will pass through the lion-guarded gates of Sutro Heights Park. This sanctuary from the hubbub of the city—with its palm trees, spectacular views, and soothing open spaces—was the site of millionaire Adolph Sutro's extravagant country mansion and sculpture garden.

Note: If you hanker for some beach walking, you can add Walk 10 to the beginning or end of Walk 11. From the start of Walk 11 in the Merrie Way parking lot, walk downhill one long block to the Cliff House and join Walk 10 in midcourse. Continue with Walk 10, visiting Ocean Beach, the Dutch Windmill, and the Beach Chalet, before returning up Point Lobos Avenue to Merrie Way. See page 140 to spot exactly where you will join Walk 10.

The walk

➤Start at the trailhead at the far end of the Merrie Way parking lot, marked by a sign for the Coastal Trail.

➤Walk along the wide dirt path bordered by flowering shrubs and wildflowers. Catch glimpses of the green-blue ocean through the Monterey pines that flank the coast. You are likely to hear sea lions barking.

➤Continue on the broad trail as it winds around this headland, which terminates in Lands End. Benches mark some of the more scenic points along this path, but all is spectacular.

➤Stop at the overlook from which you can see a buoy shaped like a giant soda can. This buoy marks Mile Rock and warns inbound ships of hazardous rocks. To the left and south of the buoy, not far from the coastline, the shipwrecked remains of the oil tankers *Lyman Stewart* and *Frank H. Buck*, both sunk in heavy fog at this spot—after being rammed by other ships—can be seen in the surf at low tide. Across the channel, you will see Point Bonita lighthouse, also designed to help ships safely enter the largest harbor on the West Coast.

➤Continue on the broad dirt trail. At Painted Rock Cliff, ascend the staircase built of railroad ties. Sixty-five steps take you up to a midway resting and camera-snapping point—the view of the Golden Gate Bridge is spectacular—and then another fifty steps take you to the top. At the base of the steps is a sign reminding hikers to stay away from the edge of the cliffs; the cliffs are unstable and people have fallen to their deaths from this area.

➤Continue on the sandy path as it leads into a shady eucalyptus grove. Crescent-shaped eucalyptus leaves litter the forest floor.

➤Continue on the trail as it grows narrower and more sinuous, meandering up and down through an open tall grass and shrub meadow. Please mind your footing when walking down the steeper sections of the trail; loose dirt can make the surface unstable.

➤The trail switches back in the opposite direction, affording great views of the Golden Gate.

➤Emerge from the hillside path onto a broad asphalt road that runs alongside the manicured greens of Lincoln Park

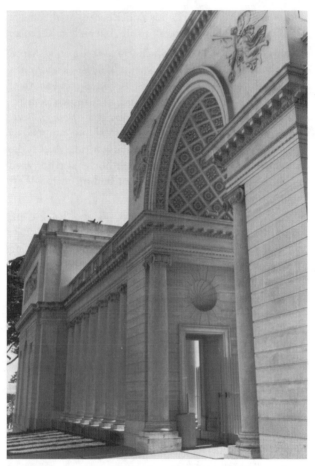

The California Palace of the Legion of Honor is one of San Francisco's fine city museums.

Municipal Golf Course. Watch out for golf cart traffic. Looking to your left you will see the back side of the California Palace of the Legion of Honor.

➤Turn left and walk up the road toward the museum.

➤At the corner of the museum, walk across Legion of Honor Drive to the sculpture created by American artist George Segal in memory of the victims of the Nazi Holocaust. This moving memorial—often strewn with flowers—is set just downslope from the left edge of the large parking lot in front of the museum.

➤Walk around the perimeter of the parking lot. Note the elegant period lampposts along the semicircular promenade, in keeping with the neoclassical museum—an exact replica of the Palais de la Legion d'Honneur in Paris—across the way. This beautifully designed overlook offers great city views. You will be able to see such landmarks—from left to right—as the Transamerica Pyramid; the bold, dark Bank of America; the University of San Francisco campus; and the University of California-San Francisco Medical Center at the base of Mount Parnassus.

➤Walk up the promenade to the entrance of the museum, past the formal flower beds, also in keeping with the French character of this majestic building. Walk along the colonnade of the outer courtyard.

The statue in the center of the colonnade is an original cast of French sculptor Auguste Rodin's *The Thinker,* its toe rubbed shiny by many an admiring schoolchild. Inside the palace is one of the world's most extensive collections of Rodin's sculptures, surely a good reason to visit this excellent museum.

Besides its Rodins, the museum holds significant collections representing the art of ancient Egypt and Rome; European painting, sculpture, and decorative arts from medieval times to the mid-20th century; and the graphic arts. The museum's Achenbach Foundation for Graphic Arts collection includes more than 70,000 prints, drawings, and illustrated books, making it one of the largest of its kind in the United States.

➤Upon leaving the museum, take an immediate left and walk down a dirt path to a set of concrete stairs. Descend the stairs, cross the driveway that runs beside the museum, and take a left into the parking lot just beyond.

➤Walk to the end of the parking lot, and there, at the sign marking the entrance to the Golden Gate National Recreation Area, take the dirt path and walk down a railroad-tie stairway leading off to the right.

➤The path curves through a shady glen and through what, at some times of the year, is a forest of 6- to 7-foot-high wild fennel plants. Other paths lead downhill from the main path; stay on the level main path.

➤Emerge at the edge of the broad oval parking lot serving Fort Miley, and walk along its perimeter for a sweeping view of the ocean, the Marin Headlands, and on a clear day, Point Reyes Peninsula up the coast. At the western edge of the lot, you will find a memorial to the USS *San Francisco* and the men who died on the cruiser in the Battle of Guadalcanal in November 1942. Made from the battle-scarred bridge of the ship, the memorial bears eloquent witness to that desperate battle.

➤Continue on the shady trail along the edge of the lot to El Camino Del Mar. Walk 1 block on El Camino Del Mar to Point Lobos Avenue.

➤Cross Point Lobos to the entrance to Sutro Heights Park, flanked by two stone lions, on the opposite corner. Walk into the park along a broad gravel promenade lined with palm trees, Monterey pines, eucalyptus, and fir.

The park—with its formal gardens, crumbling statues, and ruins—radiates old-world charm, even mystery, an effect that Adolph Sutro no doubt strove for when he created this hilltop retreat at the end of the 19th century. Sutro was a mining engineer and oceanfront developer. He built the Cliff House and Sutro Baths and later served as San Francisco's mayor.

➤The promenade continues around the perimeter of the park, along an overlook with a grand view of the Pacific Ocean. Begin walking along the perimeter in a clockwise direction, and stop as soon as you get to the perimeter wall to look out over the great expanse southward. You will see Ocean Beach, the new apartment buildings on the site of Playland at the Beach, and even farther to the south, Fort Funston and the suburb of Pacifica.

➤As you continue around the perimeter, you will see the foundations for Sutro's mansion and garden overlook and will find several ways up from all sides of this picturesque stone structure. We suggest taking the rough steps that look as if they had been carved out of the bedrock; these will lead you to the top of the parapet, where you can enjoy breathtaking views.

➤Descend from the parapet via any of the descents and continue your clockwise ramble along the promenade. On your right, you will pass a small white gazebo and a sign describing the extensive flower beds planted by Sutro. These magnificent gardens required a staff of ten gardeners just to maintain them.

➤Turn left as you rejoin the central promenade, and exit the park the same way you entered it.

➤Cross Point Lobos Avenue at the light, and walk downhill along Point Lobos until you reach Merrie Way and the parking lot where you started this walk.

walk 12

Pacific Heights and Japantown

    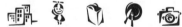

General location: Northeastern San Francisco.

Special attractions: Shopping districts, cafés and restaurants, urban landscapes, varied architecture, park, Japanese culture.

Difficulty rating: Moderate, hilly, and almost entirely on sidewalks.

Distance: 2.5 miles.

Estimated time: 1.25 hours.

Services: Restaurants, restrooms.

Restrictions: Not wheelchair accessible. A few hills are so steep that steps have been added to make climbing easier; there

Pacific Heights and Japantown

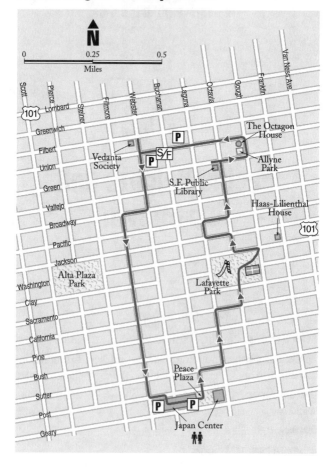

are a few dirt pathways in Lafayette Park. Dogs must be leashed—except in Lafayette Park's dog-running area—and their droppings picked up.

For more information: Contact the San Francisco Convention and Visitors Bureau.

Getting started: This walk begins at the corner of Union and Buchanan Streets.

(1) For freeway exits into San Francisco from the East Bay or the San Francisco Peninsula, refer to "Meet San Francisco" earlier in this book. From the intersection of Market, Ninth, Hayes, and Larkin Streets near the Civic Center, veer left onto Hayes and go 3 blocks. Turn right onto Franklin Street and go about 1.5 miles to Union Street. Turn left onto Union and go 4 blocks to Buchanan.

(2) From the Golden Gate Bridge, continue on U.S. Highway 101 South and veer right onto the Downtown/Lombard turnoff. Drive 7 blocks on Lombard Street, turn right onto Buchanan Street, and go 3 blocks to Union Street.

On-street parking is extremely scarce in this neighborhood. The two garages closest to the start of this walk are California Parking at 1910 Union between Laguna and Buchanan Streets, and Union Street Plaza at 2001 Union between Buchanan and Webster Streets.

Public transportation: Buses 41 and 45 of the San Francisco Municipal Railway (Muni) run along Union Street; bus 22 stops at Union and Fillmore; buses 42, 47, and 49 stop at the corner of Union and Van Ness, 5 blocks from Buchanan Street. Contact Muni for information about schedules, fares, and accessibility.

Overview: This pleasant walk leads you through the eastern half of San Francisco's most affluent, mansion-studded neighborhood, along some of the city's most appealing shopping streets, and into the rich culture of Japantown.

Unlike some of San Francisco's other unique neighborhoods, Pacific Heights can never be mistaken for a small town. This wealthy district radiates urbanity. On its steep and serene streets, you will encounter astonishing feats of residential architecture, whether they be private Victorian mansions or elegant neoclassical apartment houses.

Affluence breeds good shopping, and the two lively retail streets you visit on this walk—Union and Fillmore—offer many unique shops catering to discriminating tastes. You will also find plenty of great places to eat; we always stop at Patisserie Delanghe on Fillmore at Sutter, where famished walkers can refuel on pear-almond tarts, flaky croissants, and espresso.

As you walk down Fillmore, you will pass into still another distinctive neighborhood, the district known as Japantown. Many of San Francisco's Japanese citizens settled here, in the city's "Western Addition," after the 1906 earthquake and fire. And today, the Japanese Cultural and Trade Center on Post Street, with its many shops and restaurants, serves as a focal point for the city's thriving Japanese community.

San Francisco firefighters managed to stop the great fire of 1906 at Van Ness Avenue, thus preserving many of the fine Victorian homes—large and small—of the Western Addition and Pacific Heights. As you climb back into Pacific Heights, you will encounter some of the city's finest restored Victorians on the border between the two districts.

Finally, this walk offers you—at the highest point in Pacific Heights—lovely, 4-block Lafayette Park, with its palm trees and rolling lawns. Then, having soaked up a little nature, you just may be ready—as you descend to Union Street—to step back into the urban fray.

The walk

➤Start at the corner of Union and Buchanan Streets, facing west. Walk along Union for 1 block to Webster Street.

Union Street between Gough and Steiner Streets is one of San Francisco's most chic shopping districts, crowded with a dizzying array of antique, interior design, clothing, and art emporiums, plus an enticing bunch of excellent restaurants, bakeries, and coffee houses.

➤Turn right onto Webster and go 1 block to the corner of Webster and Filbert.

At 2963 Webster, you will encounter a San Francisco landmark, the outrageous East-meets-West confection built for the Vedanta Society in 1905 by architect Joseph Leonard. Feast your eyes on this architectural extravaganza with its bulbous Asian appurtenances and Victorian gingerbread.

➤Walk back up Webster to Union. Cross Union and climb up Webster for 3 blocks to Broadway. Between Vallejo and Broadway, steps cut into the sidewalk help mitigate Webster's steepness.

You are now entering the tony residential district known as Pacific Heights. Keep an eye out for spectacular mansions and elegant apartment houses in a variety of architectural styles.

➤Turn right onto Broadway and walk 1 block to Fillmore Street, passing the Schools of the Sacred Heart, housed in three handsome historic mansions at 2200, 2222, and 2252 Broadway.

The western part of Pacific Heights—straight ahead on Broadway—is filled with extraordinarily expensive homes and even more mansions, many of them on the scale of the ones you just passed. You may want to make a note to return another day to explore the area bounded by Broadway and

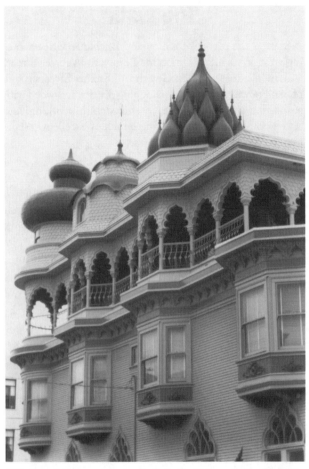

This remarkable structure was built for the Vedanta Society in 1905 and still serves as the society's monastery.

Jackson, Fillmore, and Lyon Streets. From the corner of Fillmore and Lyon, you will be able to descend the rather grand Lyon Street steps to meet up again with Union Street.

➤Turn left onto Fillmore—after stopping to take in a sweeping view of the bay—and walk down Fillmore for 8 blocks.

This stretch of Fillmore is another of San Francisco's exciting shopping districts. Here you will find all manner of specialty stores, from hat and vintage clothing shops to French patisseries to high-end purveyors of fashion and furniture.

➤Just before crossing Bush Street, look left along Bush to see a row of Victorians—at numbers 2115, 2117, 2119, and 2121 Bush—with false fronts elegantly outlined against the sky.

➤Proceed 2 blocks along Fillmore to Post Street, cross Post, and turn left. You have now entered San Francisco's Japantown neighborhood.

➤Just one building beyond the entrance to the Kabuki 8 multiplex of theaters at 1881 Post, you will find the entrance to the Kinokuniya Building, 1825 Post, one part of the Japanese Cultural and Trade Center, also known as the Japan Center. Enter the Kinokuniya Building and ascend its central stairway.

The Japan Center is one of San Francisco's cultural treasures and the heart of Japantown. Some of the center's restaurants offer the traditional Japanese style of dining, with guests seated on tatami mats at low tables. Many offer sushi or a simple menu of large bowls of noodles served quickly—just the ticket before a movie at the Kabuki 8.

Most of the Japan Center's shops focus on traditional Japanese arts and crafts. There are stores that sell Japanese prints, paper lamps, kimonos, and antique furniture. On a recent visit, we spotted a nursery that specializes in bonsai

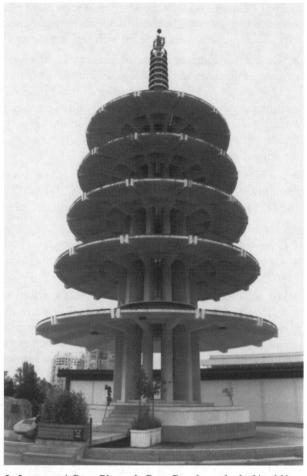

In Japantown's Peace Plaza, the Peace Pagoda marks the friendship between the United States and Japan.

trees. The center even features a Japanese-language bookstore and Japanese baths, and the National Japanese American Historical Society makes its home here.

➤At the top of the stairway, turn left and walk through a passageway that leads to the adjacent building, the Kintetsu Building.

➤Pass through the Kintetsu Building to its exit onto the open-air Peace Plaza, noted for its Peace Pagoda. The multi-tiered pagoda was presented in friendship to the people of the United States by the people of Japan in 1968.

➤Exit the Peace Plaza onto Post Street. Cross Post and walk 1 block through a walking mall of Japanese-inspired architecture. The mall is actually a block of Buchanan Street.

➤At the corner of Sutter and Buchanan Streets, cross Sutter and turn right, walking 1 block on Sutter to Laguna Street. Take a left onto Laguna.

➤The 1800 block of Laguna features—on both sides of the street—a famous and photogenic group of Victorian homes.

The beautiful Victorian at numbers 1827 and 1829 Laguna—built in 1889—sports a plaque honoring its varied history. The house's first owner, a German immigrant, was a prominent gold-rush pioneer and river pilot. A Japanese family purchased the home in the 1930s, but in a miscarriage of justice, they were interned by the U.S. government during the anti-Japanese hysteria of World War II. During the war, their home became a house of ill-repute operated by a famous San Francisco madam.

➤Continue up Laguna to California Street. Take a right onto California. Check out the spectacular row of Victorians—handsomely painted, and each different from the next—across the street, between numbers 2018 and 2026 California.

➤At the corner of California and Octavia Streets, turn left, crossing California and continuing up Octavia for 1 block.

Notice the enormous house on the corner of California and Octavia, at 1990 California, with its tower and cupola. Handsome mansions like this one—and the many stylish apartment buildings in the neighborhood—underscore the wealth and restrained good taste of the Pacific Heights district.

➤Octavia Street runs into Lafayette Park at Sacramento Street. Cross Sacramento, and pass between the set of palm trees flanking the entrance to the park. Continue straight ahead, up to the crest of the park crowned with cypress, eucalyptus, and palm trees. Lafayette Park is popular with dog lovers; it has an official dog-running area where you can take your dog off its leash.

➤At the crown of the hill, take the path that leads to the right and passes above the tennis courts. At this point, with the city out of sight, it is easy to feel as if you were in the middle of a vast natural area deep in the countryside, instead of in a 4-block park surrounded by a dense urban neighborhood.

➤Once you can see the streets below, note the row of striking Queen Anne homes on Gough Street off to your right. Head toward the far corner of the park, to the intersection of Washington and Gough Streets.

➤After descending the steps leading out of the park, turn left and walk 1 block along Washington, noting the enormous private residences—some of which have parklike grounds, an extreme luxury in this crowded city.

Note also the grand rose-colored apartment building, at 2006 Washington, with its spectacular entranceway and formal garden. The immense French-style mansion at 2080 Washington was built by George Applegarth, the architect

of interest

The Haas-Lilienthal House

As you walk through eastern Pacific Heights, you may want to make a slight detour from our route. Venture 1 block east of the corner of Washington and Gough to visit that extraordinary Queen Anne pile, the Haas-Lilienthal House. Situated at 2007 Franklin Street, this historic house is operated as a museum by the Foundation for San Francisco's Architectural Heritage. The museum—a marvelously preserved emblem of Pacific Heights' grand Victorian past—is open to the public on a limited basis. Call to schedule a tour.

The Haas-Lilienthal House was built in 1886. Like its neighbors throughout Pacific Heights, it escaped the 1906 fire because the city's fire brigades were able to stop the conflagration at Van Ness Avenue. The house's beautifully preserved interior—many of the furnishings are original—reflects the taste of William Haas and his descendants. Though this house cost nearly $20,000 to build, a hefty price in its day, other San Francisco mansions of the same period topped the $1 million mark, a testimony to the extraordinary wealth this city generated during the 19th century.

who also designed the Palace of the Legion of Honor in Lincoln Park.

▶Turn right onto Octavia and descend the hill for 1 block, through a pleasant oasis of greenery set in a brick-paved, sinuous-sided street.

▶At the corner of Octavia and Jackson, take in the view of Fort Mason, Alcatraz, and Angel Island. Then turn left onto Jackson.

Note the lovely rooftop garden at 2010 Jackson and the circular windows near the rooflines of the residences at 2045 and 2055 Jackson. The brownstone mansion at 2090 Jackson was built between 1894 and 1896.

➤At the corner of Jackson and Laguna, cross Jackson and descend the hill on Laguna for 1 block to Pacific.

➤Cross Pacific and turn right, noting the Victorians at 2023, 2021, and 2019 Pacific and the wonderful Queen Anne—with its gorgeous curved windows—at 2000 Pacific, on the corner of Octavia and Pacific. This Queen Anne sports a formal garden in its front yard, complete with roses and perfectly trimmed hedges.

➤Turn left onto Octavia, descending the hill for 3 blocks. You will pass several more fine Victorians.

➤At the corner of Octavia and Green Streets, turn left and walk one-quarter block on Green to look at the Golden Gate Valley branch of the San Francisco Public Library, the unusual neoclassical building at 1801 Green.

➤Return to the corner of Octavia and Green and continue on Green 1 block to Gough Street.

➤Turn left onto Gough and descend 1 block to Union Street. You will pass Allyne Park and then the Octagon House at 2645 Gough.

The Octagon House, built in 1857, was an offspring of the ideas of Orson Fowler, who proposed that octagonal houses were conducive to better, more healthy living. Run as a museum and open to the public, the Octagon is a project of the National Society of Colonial Dames. Call the Octagon for more information. Another octagonal house, used as a private residence, can be found on Russian Hill (see Walk 4).

➤Turn left onto Union and walk 3 blocks to the corner of Union and Buchanan and the end of this walk.

walk 13

The Castro District and Noe Valley

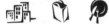

General location: In central San Francisco, below Twin Peaks, at the southwestern end of Market Street, about 2 miles southwest of Union Square.

Special attractions: Urban landscapes and vistas, neighborhood shopping districts, cafés and restaurants, varied architecture, hill climbing.

Difficulty rating: Somewhat difficult, with steep hills and stairways; entirely on sidewalks and stairways.

Distance: 4 miles.

Estimated time: 2 hours.

Services: Restaurants.

The Castro District and Noe Valley

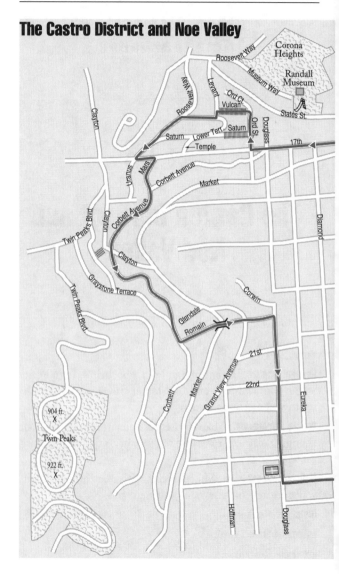

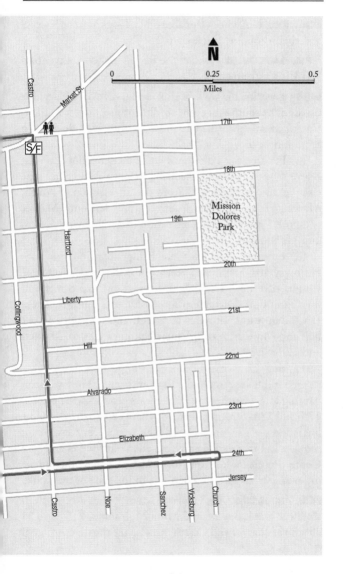

Restrictions: Not wheelchair accessible. Dogs must be leashed and their droppings picked up.

For more information: Contact the San Francisco Convention and Visitors Bureau.

Getting started: This walk begins at Harvey Milk Plaza, located at the southwest corner of the intersection of Market, Castro, and 17th Streets, 2 miles southwest of downtown San Francisco.

(1) For freeway exits into San Francisco from the East Bay or the San Francisco Peninsula, refer to "Meet San Francisco" earlier in this book. From the intersection of Ninth, Market, Hayes, and Larkin Streets, turn left onto Market and go 1.5 miles to the intersection of Market with Castro and 17th Streets.

(2) From the Golden Gate Bridge, continue on U.S. Highway 101 South and veer right onto the Downtown/Lombard turnoff. Drive 1 block on Lombard Street and turn right onto Divisadero Street. Drive 2 miles to where Divisadero turns into Castro Street, and then go another half-mile on Castro to the intersection of Castro, Market, and 17th Streets.

Parking in this neighborhood is a great challenge. On-street parking is scarce and is time-restricted. The two small parking lots near the start of the walk—on Castro between 17th and 18th Streets and on 18th between Castro and Collingwood streets—are metered for 2 hours every day except Sunday. Limited parking is also available at Market and Noe Center Public Parking on Noe Street. We recommend taking public transportation or a taxi to the start of this walk.

Public transportation: San Francisco Municipal Railway (Muni) streetcar line F, bus 24, and Muni Metro lines K, L, and M all stop at Market and Castro Streets. See the description of the historic F streetcars in Walk 1, Downtown. Contact Muni for information about schedules, fares, and accessibility.

Overview: This invigorating walk takes you into three distinct—and distinctive—San Francisco neighborhoods. First, from the corner of Castro and Market Streets, you climb into the Upper Castro and lower Twin Peaks residential areas. Here you will encounter the garden-lined and very steep Vulcan Street stairs. This neighborhood is notable for its eclectic mix of architectural styles and its maze of curvy streets, so unlike the grid that overlays the rest of San Francisco. Walking these winding streets—rarely visited by tourists—underscores San Francisco's rich diversity and the quality of life its citizens enjoy.

This walk next leads you into Noe Valley, currently one of San Francisco's hottest neighborhoods. For many years a quiet, family-oriented district, Noe Valley is a favored address these days for the city's young and affluent. Hidden by a hill from downtown San Francisco, Noe Valley seems like a village in a valley, recently gentrified perhaps, but still very much a small town. For better and worse, Noe Valley is changing: Its shopping district—along 24th Street—grows ever more sophisticated, its excellent restaurants are garnering accolades citywide, and real estate prices are skyrocketing. Book fanciers especially will love Noe Valley; there are several fine used and new bookstores within blocks of each other along 24th.

The final neighborhood on this walk is the Castro District, which, unlike the Upper Castro, is rarely quiet. The Castro, with its overwhelmingly gay population, is an important neighborhood for San Francisco's identity. More than most American cities, San Francisco is truly diverse, especially in terms of ethnicity and sexual orientation. San

Franciscans celebrate, take pride in, and are truly comfortable with that diversity. This accepting attitude is one of the most distinctive and beautiful things about this city.

Our walk ends, as it began, in Harvey Milk Plaza across from the historic Castro Theater. Harvey Milk—San Francisco's first openly gay city supervisor—was tragically assassinated, along with the city's mayor, George Moscone, on November 27, 1978. Every year on November 27, San Franciscans bearing candles march from the Castro to City Hall as a memorial to the two men.

The walk

➤Start at Harvey Milk Plaza, the small brick-paved plaza located at the three-way intersection of Market, Castro, and 17th Streets. On this plaza is the main entrance to the Castro/Market Muni Metro station; escalators lead from the plaza down to the underground station.

➤Cross Market Street at the light, and just beyond Market, turn left onto the sidewalk that parallels 17th Street. Seventeenth is not well-marked at this point, but continue up the sidewalk and you will soon see a street sign confirming that you are, indeed, on 17th.

➤Walk uphill on 17th for 4 blocks to Ord Street. The last two blocks are fairly steep.

➤Turn right onto Ord, a quiet enclave of bungalows and Victorians. Walk about 1 block on Ord, past the Saturn Street stairs, to the Vulcan Street stairs. Before climbing the stairs, look toward the end of Ord and upward to see the rocky outcropping of Corona Heights, an island of wild hillside rising above the Castro District.

➤Turn left onto the Vulcan Street stairs and climb the steps—about 215 in all—to the top. When you have climbed about 55 steps, a second stairway will branch off to the left. Stay on the right-hand set of stairs.

In this quiet ravine in the bosom of the city, gardens flourish. These lush and quirky labors-of-love feature flowers, herbs, bamboo hedges, berry bushes, palm trees, and a wild variety of exotic plants. Friends who live in this neighborhood say that many houses have beautiful private gardens in their backyards, that some residents raise ducks and chickens, and that bold raccoons have been known to pass through cat doors to dine from a pet's food dish left on the kitchen floor.

➤At the top of the Vulcan stairs, turn left onto Levant Street and go a partial block to Lower Terrace.

➤Turn right onto Lower Terrace and walk uphill 1 block to Roosevelt Way. You will find a wide variety of architectural styles along here, from Mission bungalows to Victorians to basic San Francisco flats, with the requisite bay windows and garage underneath.

➤Turn left onto Roosevelt and walk 2 mercifully level blocks back to 17th Street. Far up ahead you will see San Francisco's Twin Peaks—904 feet and 922 feet above sea level—and Sutro Tower atop nearby Mount Sutro. This enormous antenna, which many consider an appalling eyesore, transmits radio, television, and microwave signals throughout the Bay Area.

➤Cross 17th Street at the stop sign. There is a small grocery on this corner, your last chance to buy refreshments until you reach Noe Valley, about 1 mile farther on.

➤Turn left onto 17th and walk downhill 1 short block to Mars Street.

➤Turn right onto Mars and walk 1 block to Corbett Street, where Mars dead-ends.

➤Cross Corbett, turn right, and walk uphill on Corbett. On your left, near the street sign marking the intersection of Mono and Corbett Streets, you will pass Twin Peaks East Association Community Park, with its benches and planted hillside—a welcome resting spot.

➤Where Corbett meets Clayton Street, turn left and walk along Clayton a short distance until you reach a crosswalk.

➤Cross Clayton, and continue straight ahead on the continuation of Corbett as it winds upward through the lower part of Twin Peaks, with its 1960s multi-unit structures built to take advantage of spectacular views of the city and the bay.

➤Continue on Corbett as it intersects Graystone Terrace and Glendale Street. Peek through the fences along Corbett for some fine vistas of Noe Valley, downtown San Francisco, and the Mission District.

➤When you reach Romain Street, turn left onto Romain and walk downhill 1 block past a series of delightful 1930s Spanish-style stucco bungalows adorned with small flower gardens and carefully manicured hedges and trees.

➤At the bottom of this block of Romain Street, cross Market Street on the pedestrian bridge. From the bridge, take in the sweeping views of downtown San Francisco and the East Bay.

➤Continue walking downhill on Romain for another 2 blocks.

➤Turn right onto Douglass Street and walk 6 blocks to 24th Street. As you cross 23rd Street, glance up and down 23rd to see clusters of Victorians.

➤Turn left onto 24th Street and walk 5 blocks to Church Street.

On 24th, between Diamond and Church Streets, lies the busy shopping area of the Noe Valley neighborhood. This street features the cafés and restaurants, bookstores and bakeries, gourmet food shops, wine merchants, and other small businesses that make up a real working neighborhood. Although there are a few chain coffee houses, most of Noe Valley's businesses are one-of-a-kind, and many are housed in old Victorians. If you need a pick-me-up after your hill-climbing, this is just the place.

➤Cross to the opposite side of 24th Street and walk back 3 blocks to Castro Street.

➤Turn right onto Castro and walk 3 steep blocks to Alvarado Street at the crest of the hill. Many beautifully painted and lovingly maintained Victorians line this stretch of Castro. At each street corner, look up and down the cross streets for even more Victorian gazing.

➤Continue on Castro and descend 6 blocks to 19th Street and the heart of "the Castro," one of the best-known gay neighborhoods in the United States.

The Castro's bustling commercial district starts at 19th and Castro. Here you will find vintage clothing, antique, and home furnishing stores as well as cafés, bars, and restaurants. On the right side of Castro, you will see the large neon sign for the Castro Theater, a neighborhood landmark built in 1922 and one of the last grand movie theaters in San Francisco.

The Castro Theater shows a strong program of excellent foreign and classic movies, and—keeping alive a venerable cinematic tradition—it nightly features music from its Wurlitzer pipe organ. Self-described as the "cathedral of Cinema," the Castro is ". . . an ornate Spanish Colonial confection . . . [and] a mishmash of architectural genres mixing an elaborate Spanish Colonial facade with interior murals and fixtures that draw on Asian, Arab, and Art Deco influences."

➤Continue past the Castro Theater to the corner of 17th, Castro, and Market Streets. Cross Castro to return to Harvey Milk Plaza and the end of this walk.

walk 14

Mission Murals

General location: In central San Francisco, off Mission Street about 2.5 miles south of Union Square.

Special attractions: Colorful murals, distinctive neighborhood, restaurants.

Difficulty rating: Easy, flat, and entirely on sidewalks.

Distance: 2 miles.

Estimated time: 1 hour.

Services: Restaurants.

Restrictions: Wheelchair accessible. Dogs must be leashed and their droppings picked up. The murals in this neighborhood are copyrighted works of art. Feel free to photograph them for your personal use, but note that photos of

Mission Murals

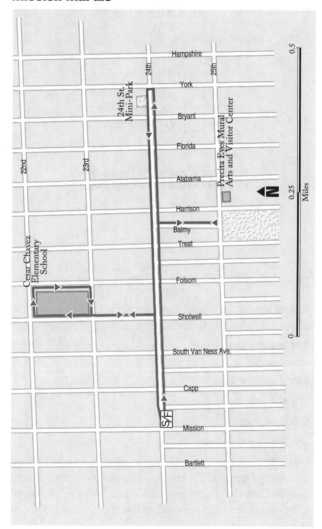

the murals cannot be reproduced except with written permission from the muralist(s). If you wish to obtain permission, call Precita Eyes Mural Arts Center.

For more information: Contact the San Francisco Convention and Visitors Bureau or Precita Eyes Mural Arts Center.

Getting started: This walk begins at the corner of Mission and 24th Streets.

(1) For freeway exits into San Francisco from the East Bay or the San Francisco Peninsula, refer to "Meet San Francisco" earlier in this book. From the intersection of Ninth and Howard Streets—2 blocks south of the intersection of Market, Ninth, Larkin, and Hayes Streets—drive east on Howard for 4 blocks until Howard merges into South Van Ness Avenue. Continue southward on South Van Ness for 1.25 miles to 24th Street. Turn right onto 24th Street, and go 2 blocks to Mission Street.

(2) From the Golden Gate Bridge, continue on U.S. Highway 101 South and veer right onto the Downtown/Lombard turnoff. Drive about 1 mile on Lombard Street to Van Ness Avenue. Turn right onto Van Ness and drive 1.75 miles to Market Street. Cross Market and continue on South Van Ness for 1.5 miles. Turn right onto 24th Street and go 2 blocks to Mission Street.

There are no parking garages close by in this neighborhood, but on-street parking is available on 24th and its side streets.

Public transportation: Buses 14 and 49 of the San Francisco Municipal Railway (Muni) and all trains of the Bay Area Rapid Transit (BART) system stop at 24th and Mission Streets. Muni bus 26 stops at Valencia Street and Mission, 2 blocks from the start of this walk. Buses 14 and 26 and all BART trains are wheelchair accessible; bus 49 is not.

Contact Muni or BART for information about schedules, fares, and accessibility.

Overview: Twenty-fourth Street in the Mission District, like many of San Francisco's neighborhoods, has the feel of a small town. Most of what a neighborhood needs can be found along this tree-lined stretch between Mission and York Streets: vegetable and grocery stores, *panaderias* (bakeries), restaurants, meat markets, a hardware store, bookstores, a record/CD store—with the largest collection of Latino music in San Francisco—art galleries, and numerous gift shops.

And 24th Street has something that no other neighborhood in the city offers: an amazing array of beautiful, well-crafted, and often thought-provoking murals depicting themes of importance to the artists and the residents of the neighborhood. There are more than 80 murals in the Mission District, and this walk samples a representative group of them along 24th Street.

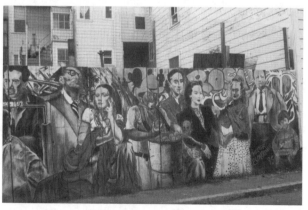

Balmy Alley is lined by nearly 30 murals on fences and garage doors, including this one by artist Hector Escarraman, entitled Icons of Mexican Art.

The Murals of Balmy Alley

The murals on the back fences and garage doors of this quiet alley have been created over three decades, from 1971 to the present. Some show the weathered charm of their many years; others are so worn that they are barely discernible; and still others are bright and new.

Some of the murals are lighthearted, and many reflect pride in Latino culture. One honors cultural icons like the great Mexican muralist Diego Rivera—one of the founders of the Mexican mural movement—and his wife, the painter Frida Kahlo. Another shows the Mexican film stars Cantinflas, Dolores Del Rio, and Tin Tan. The mural *Low Riding Madness* celebrates low-rider culture—and it even includes a low-rider bicyclist. *Latino Pride* is a collaboration between a spray-can artist and a muralist using traditional acrylic paints.

Other murals on Balmy Alley deal with more painful subjects. One political mural shows mothers holding photos of family members "disappeared" by the death squads. Another, *Indigenous Eyes: War or Peace,* makes a statement about Central American politics and history. Look closely at this mural to see the haunting reflections in the eyes. *We Remember* is a memorial to those who have died of AIDS.

The walk

➤Start at the corner of 24th and Mission Streets, in front of the McDonald's restaurant on the southeast corner. This is probably the only McDonald's in the world covered with a vibrant mural created by neighborhood kids.

➤Face 24th Street, turn right, and begin your stroll into the 24th Street business district. Keep your eyes peeled for murals; there are usually several on every block.

➤Walk 5.5 blocks to Balmy Alley a street only 1 block long that resembles a pedestrian walkway. Balmy Alley has nearly 30 murals, the highest concentration in the Mission.

➤Turn right into Balmy Alley, walk to the end, and then return to 24th Street.

➤Turn right onto 24th Street and walk for one-half block to Harrison Street.

On this corner, at "La Gallinita" Belmar Meat Market, is a mural of two mythic Mexican figures: Popocatepetl, a warrior, and Ixtaccihuatl, the daughter of the emperor. Their love was ill-fated, and as Ixtaccihuatl lay dying, Popocatepetl swept her away. Transformed into mountains, the lovers lie side by side outside Mexico City, together forever. These figures appear in many Mission murals, for this is a very popular Mexican love story.

➤Continue on 24th Street one-half block to the Precita Eyes Mural Arts and Visitor Center at 2981 24th Street.

This center conducts mural tours and workshops, and the friendly folks behind the counter provide Mission District cultural and business information. Feel free to stop in to look at the mural-covered walls, check out the colorful mural postcards, or pick up a map that identifies the 84 murals in the Mission District.

➤Continue on 24th another half block to Alabama Street. The Mexican bakery on this corner—Panaderia Dominguez (La Flor de Jalisco)—is adorned with *trompe l'oeil* roof tiles over its windows as well as heroic figures on its exterior walls.

➤Continue on 24th for one-half block, and stop to look at the mid-block mural at China Books and Periodicals, *A Bountiful Harvest*. China Books commissioned this mural in the style of Chinese social realism—except that this classic Chinese harvest scene includes people of many races.

➤Continue on 24th another half block to Florida. On this corner is the intense and powerful mural *500 Años de Resistencia* ("500 Years of Resistance"), painted by Isaías Mata on two sides of St. Peter's Church in 1993. This mural depicts the survival of native cultures despite the invasion of the American continents by Europeans.

➤Continue on 24th 1 block to Bryant. On this corner is the Galeria de la Raza.

Founded in 1970, Galeria de la Raza is one of the oldest Latino arts organizations in the United States. It offers art exhibitions, multimedia presentations, and educational activities related to Chicano/Latino art. It often sponsors a mural on the Bryant Street side of its building to advertise new exhibitions. One day we witnessed two muralists working hard to complete their mural before a gallery opening at the end of the week.

➤Continue on 24th for 1 block to York Street. The St. Francis Fountain and Candy Store has been on this corner since 1918. This old-time family-run soda fountain is known for its handmade ice cream and candy.

➤Cross 24th to the opposite side, and look across York at the powerful mural on the side of SF Taqueria. *Las Lechugueras*, painted in 1983 by Juana Alicia, pays tribute to Mexican-American women farmworkers. It also depicts the harshness of the conditions these women must endure—including exposure to pesticides sprayed on the fields while they are working.

➤Walk back one-half block on 24th toward Mission Street.

Mid-block between York and Bryant Streets is the 24th Street Mini-Park. This park's murals, created between 1974 and 1990, were designed to teach children in the community about their Latin-American heritage.

➤Continue 1.5 blocks to Florida Street and La Palma Market, one of the last places in the Mission selling handmade tortillas. The mural on the Florida Street side of the market is an eye-catching advertisement for those tortillas.

➤Continue 5 blocks on 24th to Shotwell Street. Turn right onto Shotwell.

➤Go 2 blocks on Shotwell to 22nd Street, passing by the front entrance of the Cesar Chavez Elementary School. This school is covered with some of the most beautiful murals in the Mission, and this loop will take you around all four sides.

➤Turn right onto 22nd, go 1 block to Folsom, turn right, and walk 1 block on Folsom.

In this block of Folsom, you will pass the school playground, which is dominated by the larger-than-life mural called *Si Se Puede* ("If We Can"). Painted in vibrant reds, blues, yellows, and greens, this mural weaves in and out among the classroom windows. It is anchored by a 2-story-high portrait of Cesar Chavez—the great farmworker organizer—over the school doors.

➤Turn right onto 23rd Street and walk 1 block to Shotwell Street.

➤Turn left onto Shotwell and go 1 block to 24th.

➤Turn right onto 24th and walk 3 blocks to the corner of Mission and 24th and the end of this walk.

walk 15

Golden Gate Park

   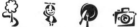

General location: In central San Francisco, about 3 miles west of Union Square.

Special attractions: Park, art and science museums, Japanese tea garden, botanical gardens, boating.

Difficulty rating: Easy, with a few moderate hills.

Distance: 3.75 miles.

Estimated time: 2 hours.

Services: Parking; restrooms; snack bar; visitor information center; bicycle, rickshaw, and boat rentals.

Restrictions: Not wheelchair accessible. Dogs must be leashed and their droppings picked up. On Sundays, John F. Kennedy Drive is closed to auto traffic; use public transportation or park on other park roadways.

Golden Gate Park

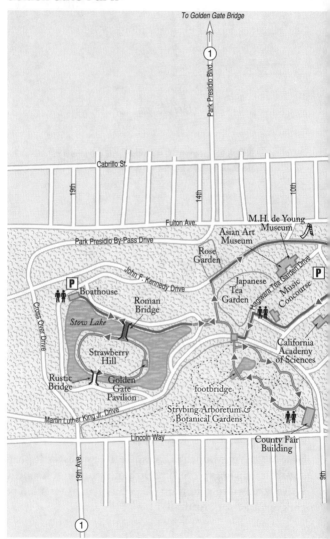

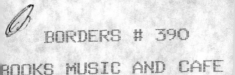

BORDERS # 390

BOOKS MUSIC AND CAFE

1144 Lake St
Oak Park, IL 60301
708-386-6927

STORE: 0390   REG: 04/69 TRAN#: 9741
SALE   03/17/2002 EMP: 00376

TIME OUT SAN FRANCISCO-E04
    6728931   QP T   14.95
WALKING SAN FRANCISCO
    6198642   QP T   10.95

           Subtotal   25.90
           ILLINOIS 8.75%   2.27
2 Items   Total   28.17
           VISA   28.17
ACCT # /S XXXXXXXXXXXX8151
              AUTH: 048103
NAME: NELSON/MARY

CUSTOMER COPY

03/17/2002 01:41PM

THANK YOU FOR SHOPPING AT BORDERS
PLEASE ASK ABOUT OUR SPECIAL EVENTS

Visit our website @ www.borders.com.

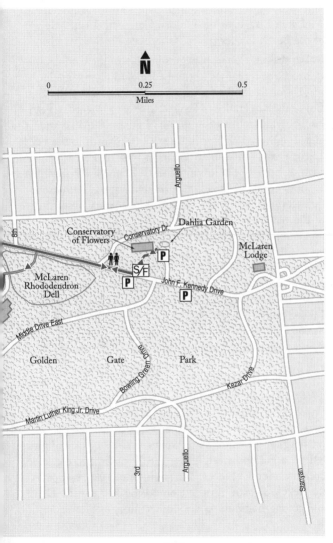

For more information: Contact the San Francisco Convention and Visitors Bureau, Golden Gate Park headquarters at McLaren Lodge, or the Golden Gate Park Visitor Center at the Beach Chalet.

Getting started: This walk begins in front of the Conservatory of Flowers, near the eastern edge of Golden Gate Park.

(1) For freeway exits into San Francisco from the East Bay or the San Francisco Peninsula, refer to "Meet San Francisco" earlier in this book. From Interstate 80 West and/or U.S. Highway 101 North, take US 101 North to the Fell/Laguna exit. Drive about 1.5 miles west on Fell Street. At Stanyan Street, Fell turns into John F. Kennedy Drive, which is one of Golden Gate Park's main roadways. Continue one-quarter mile on John F. Kennedy Drive to the Conservatory of Flowers.

Coming from the San Francisco Peninsula, you can also take I-280 North to the Golden Gate Bridge/19th Avenue exit just beyond Daly City. Continue on California Highway 1 North for almost 5 miles, over Junipero Serra Boulevard and 19th Avenue and through Golden Gate Park. Immediately upon exiting the park, turn right onto Fulton Street, go 3.5 blocks, and turn right onto 10th Avenue. At the next stop sign, turn left onto John F. Kennedy Drive and go one-half mile to the Conservatory of Flowers.

(2) From the Golden Gate Bridge, take the Park Presidio/19th Avenue exit and drive about 2 miles south on Park Presidio Boulevard. One block before reaching Golden Gate Park, turn right onto Cabrillo Street and then make an immediate left turn onto 14th Avenue. Drive 1 block and turn left onto Fulton Street. Cross Park Presidio and continue on Fulton for 3.5 blocks. Turn right onto 10th Avenue. At the next stop sign, turn left onto John F. Kennedy Drive and go one-half mile to the Conservatory of Flowers.

Park along John F. Kennedy Drive as close as possible to the Conservatory of Flowers, the unmistakable and grand white glass-and-wood structure.

Public transportation: Bus lines 5, 7, 21, 33, and 43 of the San Francisco Municipal Railway (Muni) stop within 1 to 5 blocks of McLaren Lodge. Contact Muni for schedules, fares, and accessibility.

Overview: Golden Gate Park—like Fisherman's Wharf, Chinatown, and the Golden Gate Bridge—is an inextricable part of the image most of us have of San Francisco. And the astonishing thing is that the actual park is even more beautiful and complex than the image could ever be.

In the 1,017 acres of Golden Gate Park, you can pursue nearly every outdoor activity, from in-line skating to lawn bowling to fly casting to horseback riding. You can wander through redwood groves, rhododendron dells, botanical gardens, or a Japanese tea garden. You can row a boat or dance to reggae or run for miles along forest paths. You can gaze at masterpieces of European and Asian art, learn about the world's fishes, or picnic in grassy meadows.

Golden Gate Park had inauspicious beginnings, at least for an open space now known for its magnificent gardens and towering trees. First chosen as the site for a great public park in 1870, this acreage consisted of sand dunes whipped by ocean winds. Civil engineer William Hammond Hall was the park's first superintendent, and in addition to surveying the park and providing much of its design, he began the long process of turning a sandy waste into a luxuriant parkland, planting beach grasses imported from France, lupine, and barley to stabilize the dunes. The park's second hero, Scottish garden designer John McLaren, carried out Hall's design over a nearly sixty-year career, creating the park we know today.

Our walk leads you through a representative sampling of the park's attractions, from the Conservatory of Flowers to the museums surrounding the Music Concourse, from the Strybing Arboretum and Botanical Gardens to the tranquil waters of Stow Lake. This stroll through the eastern half of the park is meant only to suggest the depth and breadth of the place. Many San Franciscans have spent a lifetime exploring this expanse of greenery. Find your own favorite places. Return again and again.

The walk

➤Start in front of the Conservatory of Flowers on John F. Kennedy Drive.

The conservatory, a Victorian marvel of wood and glass built in 1878, is the oldest building in Golden Gate Park. The conservatory was heavily damaged by a winter storm in

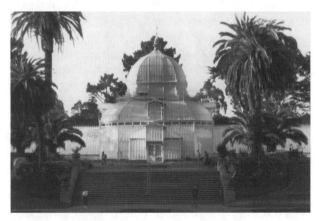

The Conservatory of Flowers is a regal presence on the eastern edge of Golden Gate Park.

1995 and has been closed to the public since then. Restoration costs are estimated at $12 million, and a fundraising program is well under way.

Before starting out, take in the colorful formal gardens in front of the conservatory and the gorgeous dahlia garden to its right.

➤Once you have finished exploring, return to John F. Kennedy Drive. Use the pedestrian tunnel to cross this often busy street and then proceed to your right along John F. Kennedy Drive.

➤After about one-quarter mile, you will come upon a large wooden sign marking the entrance into the John McLaren Rhododendron Dell. Turn left into the dell onto the broad path that leads away from John F. Kennedy Drive into a verdant grove. Soon you will pass agapanthus and rhododendron bushes and expanses of raspberries.

➤Continue on this trail, bearing always to the right wherever the path forks, until you emerge into the parking area for the museums and gardens surrounding the Music Concourse.

This remarkable complex is made up of the California Academy of Sciences building—which includes Steinhart Aquarium, Morrison Planetarium, and the Natural History Museum—and across the concourse, the M. H. de Young Museum and the Asian Art Museum. Just beyond the Asian Art Museum lies the Japanese Tea Garden.

➤Bearing left, walk along the perimeter of the Music Concourse, passing by the Academy of Sciences building. Here, in the Music Concourse, with its rows of plane and palm trees, you may happen upon a formal concert—or an impromptu guitar fest, as we did on one visit.

➤Walk behind the bandstand, where you will find restrooms and a snack bar.

of interest

Culture and Science

Not just for those eager to immerse themselves in the great outdoors, Golden Gate Park is home to some of San Francisco's finest cultural and scientific institutions. Surrounding the Music Concourse, three museums—plus an aquarium, a planetarium, and a Japanese tea garden—offer a smorgasbord of attractions.

If you are hungry for the visual arts, visit the M. H. de Young Memorial Museum. Here you will find a strong permanent collection that ranges over most of the world's continents and nearly every artistic style and period. The de Young also brings superb traveling exhibits—featuring masters like Monet and Van Gogh—to the Bay Area.

Under the same roof, the Asian Art Museum of San Francisco covers those regions of the world that the de Young does not. From China to Japan, India to Korea, the Asian Art Museum's collections reflect the rich cultures of Asia. And the museum features a never-ending array of lectures, literature readings, films and videos, demonstrations, and concerts.

Across the Music Concourse stands the California Academy of Sciences. Here you will discover three remarkable institutions—the Natural History Museum, the Steinhart Aquarium, and the Morrison Planetarium—devoted to interpreting various aspects of the physical universe. Kids will find these institutions—like the Exploratorium in Walk 7—wonderfully accessible, educational, and fun.

When you have had your fill of art and science, step across Hagiwara Tea Garden Drive to the front gate of the Japanese Tea Garden. Built for the 1894 California Mid-Winter Exposition, this serene garden—with its carefully crafted gates and bridge, its hills and waters based on classic rural Japanese gardens—is a great place to stop and have a cup of tea before you continue on your stroll through Golden Gate Park.

➤Cross Hagiwara Tea Garden Drive to the gate to the Japanese Tea Garden, turn left, and walk down Hagiwara Tea Garden Drive to its junction with Martin Luther King, Jr. Drive.

➤Take a right onto the sidewalk that parallels Martin Luther King, Jr. Drive.

➤After walking a short distance along Martin Luther King, Jr. Drive, you will come to a crosswalk. Cross the drive here and enter the Strybing Arboretum and Botanical Gardens through the Friend Gate.

Paradise for plant lovers, the Strybing Arboretum and Botanical Gardens are truly remarkable, and they extend far beyond the route outlined in this walk. However, if you do venture from our route, you may find it challenging to chart your way through the maze of trails and gardens. For the best experience, we recommend that you pick up the self-guided tour map available at the Strybing bookstore, which you will encounter later in this walk. Strybing also offers— free of charge—docent-led garden walks and theme tours. Call the Strybing office for times.

➤Once inside the gardens, take the pathway to your immediate left. Do not descend toward the pond straight ahead. The left-hand path leads you past the Primitive Plants Garden. Take a moment to explore—on the boardwalk loop— this fascinating grouping of plant species that have survived relatively unchanged through many thousands of years. The boardwalk brings you back to the main path.

➤Turn right and continue on the main path, generally bearing left, as it wanders through the trees.

➤The next named gardens you will encounter—on your right—are the Biblical Garden, featuring plants mentioned in the Bible, and just beyond, the Fragrance Garden, with strongly scented plants from all over the world. Walk through these gardens, savoring the sights and smells, and return to the main path. Up ahead you will see an open expanse of lawn and the San Francisco County Fair Building.

►Continue on the path to reach the fair building. Pass under the building's trellis and stop for a minute to visit the Strybing bookstore, situated in its own tiny structure.

This small but excellent bookstore features a wide selection of gardening and botanical books. An interpretive panel beside the store offers plenty of informative brochures. Across the way, the Helen Crocker Russell Library of Horticulture, with its 18,000-volume collection, is open to the public.

►Pass back under the trellis and return to the main path, bearing left onto the trail that leads along the outer edge of the central lawn. On your left, you will pass restrooms as the path curves toward a large fountain.

►Upon reaching the fountain, you will see a pond up ahead. Follow the path down to the pond. Cross the pond on a small wooden bridge. The Friend Gate will be up ahead.

Off to your left is a labyrinth of paths leading through many different plant collections and ecosystems, from a New World tropical cloud forest to a redwood forest to a "Moon Viewing" garden to a garden of California native plants. Wander these richly diverse gardens at your leisure. The self-guided tour materials will be useful here.

►When you are ready to leave the Strybing Arboretum and Botanical Gardens, return to the Friend Gate.

►Exit through the Friend Gate and cross Martin Luther King, Jr. Drive at the crosswalk. Continue straight ahead, following the asphalt path that leads into the trees.

►After passing a no-longer-used exit from the Japanese Tea Garden, veer left at the next intersection. Head uphill and away from the tea garden.

➤Climb the set of concrete stairs that leads to Stow Lake, cross the roadway that circles Stow Lake, and turn right. Stow Lake is a wonderful place for families. You will see picnickers, parents with strollers, kids gleefully feeding the ducks, and families exploring the lake by boat. Proceed counterclockwise on the broad asphalt path that leads along the shore.

➤Watch for a small roadway that veers off to the left and across a concrete bridge known as the Roman Bridge.

➤Cross the bridge and turn right onto the broad dirt trail that circles the base of Strawberry Hill, the little mountain that dominates the island in the middle of Stow Lake.

➤Follow the trail that circles the perimeter of the island. This tree-shaded path is a favorite of walkers and runners, dreamers and nature lovers. Among the attractions you will encounter along the way are the stone Rustic Bridge; the ornate Golden Gate Pavilion, a gift to San Francisco from its sister city, Taipei, Taiwan; and picturesque Huntington Falls.

➤Return to the Roman Bridge, and cross to the mainland. Turn left and walk to the Boathouse, where you will find restrooms; boat, rickshaw, and bicycle rentals; and a snack bar. You can also purchase a detailed map to Golden Gate Park at the snack bar.

The Boathouse is a great place to take a breather. Watch for rows of turtles sunning themselves on half-submerged logs; families setting off in rowboats, electric motor boats, and pedal boats; and the always-hungry gulls, geese, and ducks of Stow Lake.

➤When you are ready to move on, retrace your steps along the lakeshore and return to the asphalt path that first brought you to the lake from Friend Gate. Descend the concrete stairs, and at the bottom of the stairs—instead of turning right and returning to Martin Luther King, Jr. Drive and the Friend Gate—turn left. This path takes you around the back side of the Japanese Tea Garden and to John F. Kennedy Drive.

➤At the crosswalk, cross John F. Kennedy Drive to the park's extensive Rose Garden. Depending on the time of year, you may want to stop and smell the roses.

➤Turn right and walk along the sidewalk that parallels John F. Kennedy Drive.

Just beyond Tenth Avenue, you will pass a very appealing children's playground. This sparkling new play area offers the latest in brightly colored jungle gyms and other child-friendly equipment.

➤Return to the Conservatory of Flowers and the end of this walk.

walk 16

The Presidio

General location: In northwestern San Francisco, just southeast of the Golden Gate Bridge. Part of the Golden Gate National Recreation Area (GGNRA).

Special attractions: Natural landscapes, historical architecture.

Difficulty rating: Moderate and almost entirely on dirt paths.

Distance: 2 miles.

Estimated time: 1 hour.

Services: Parking, restrooms, visitor information center.

Restrictions: Not wheelchair accessible. Dogs must either be leashed or under voice control, depending on where you are walking in the Golden Gate National Recreation Area. In some areas, pets are even prohibited entirely to protect sensitive resources. Dog droppings must be picked up. Contact

The Presidio

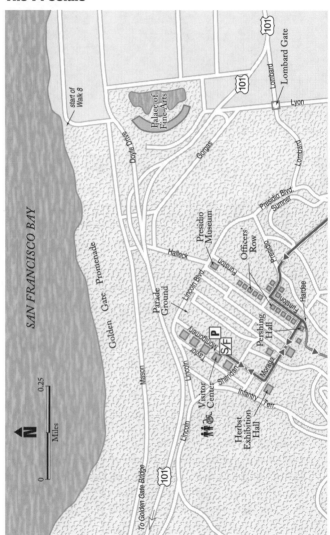

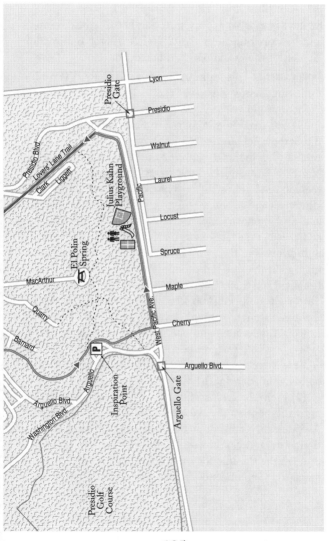

the GGNRA headquarters at Fort Mason for a listing of pet regulations.

For more information: Contact the San Francisco Convention and Visitors Bureau or the GGNRA Visitor Information Center for the Presidio of San Francisco.

Getting started: This walk begins at the GGNRA Visitor Information Center located at the Main Post parade ground in the Presidio.

(1) For freeway exits into San Francisco from the East Bay or the San Francisco Peninsula, refer to "Meet San Francisco" earlier in this book. From the intersection of Market, Ninth, Hayes, and Larkin Streets near the Civic Center, veer left onto Hayes and go 3 blocks. Turn right onto Franklin Street and go about 1.75 miles to Lombard Street. Turn left onto Lombard and go 11 blocks to Broderick Street, ending up in the left-hand lane. Just after Broderick, as the traffic curves to the right, remain on Lombard and follow the sign at the stop light to the Presidio. Go 1.5 blocks on Lombard and enter the Presidio through the Lombard Gate. Turn right onto Presidio Boulevard at the first stop sign. Continue straight through several stops—you are now on Lincoln Boulevard—and pass by the foot of the main parade ground, now a large parking lot. Turn left onto Montgomery Street and park in front of the fourth large brick building on your right. This is the visitor center.

(2) From the Golden Gate Bridge, pass through the far right toll booth and take an immediate right at the 25th Avenue exit. Turn left at the first stop sign onto Lincoln Boulevard and continue on Lincoln as it twists and turns through the Presidio for about 1.5 miles. At the foot of the main parade ground, now a large parking lot, turn right onto

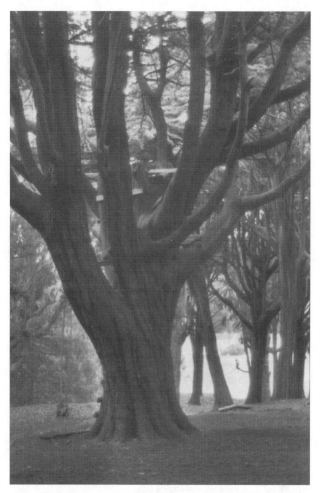

A stand of Monterey cypress shades the trail through the Presidio forest.

Montgomery Street and park in front of the fourth large brick building on your right. This is the visitor center.

Public transportation: Bus 43 of the San Francisco Municipal Railway (Muni) stops at Lombard Street and Presidio Boulevard, where you can transfer to bus 29, which stops at the corner of Lincoln and Halleck Street, a few blocks from the main parade ground and visitor center. Contact Muni for information about schedules, fares, and accessibility.

Overview: This short and gentle ramble takes you through that remarkable blend of military history and gorgeous green space that is the Presidio of San Francisco. Founded in 1776 by Spanish troops intent on colonizing the wilds of California, this outpost—then known as Presidio de San Francisco—has changed hands three times. First Spanish, then Mexican, and finally American, it retained its military character until 1994, when it passed to the National Park Service and the Presidio Trust.

A key part of the Golden Gate National Recreation Area, the Presidio is, as the National Park Service notes, "a new kind of park: one dedicated not only to preserving and protecting its resources, but also to finding solutions to environmental, cultural, and social issues of global significance." Today, the Presidio's many buildings—like those at Fort Mason, another former military facility now integrated into the GGNRA—house a wide variety of nonprofit organizations.

This walk leads you past several historic buildings on the Presidio's Main Post and through beautiful woodlands. The forest path is sparsely traveled during the week, but on almost any day, you will encounter fellow walkers, folks taking their dogs for a stroll, and joggers.

This verdant countryside, like much of San Francisco, was originally made up of sand dunes blasted by ocean winds.

The Presidio forest is the result of an ambitious tree-planting project undertaken in the late 19th century. Between 1886 and 1897, the Army planted 100,000 trees of 200 types here. The project was designed, in the words of Major W. A. Jones, "to crown the ridges, border the boundary fences and cover the areas of sand and marsh waste with a forest that will generally seem continuous, and thus appear immensely larger than it really is." Today's vast Presidio forest is dominated by three nonnative species: eucalyptus, Monterey cypress, and Monterey pine. The park service is currently engaged in bringing back many of the plants native to this landscape, and by 2010, there will be 245 acres in the Presidio devoted to native plant communities.

Much to the benefit of present-day San Franciscans, military use of the Presidio—in one of those ironies of history—has preserved this natural area, preventing the development that would undoubtedly have occurred throughout these 1,500 acres of beautifully sited and priceless real estate.

The walk

➤Start at the GGNRA Visitor Information Center on Montgomery Street at the west side of the Presidio's main parade ground. The visitor center is located in one of five identical buildings built as enlisted men's barracks in 1895–1897; two of these buildings were used to hospitalize troops injured in the Philippines during the Spanish-American War.

➤With your back to the visitor center, turn right and walk uphill to Sheridan Avenue.

➤Cross Sheridan and continue uphill 2 short blocks to Moraga Avenue and the Herbst Exhibition Hall, which features exhibits about science, culture, and history.

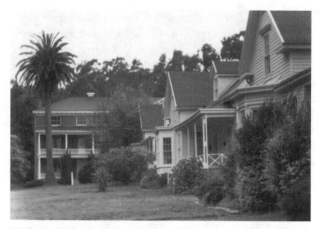

These Civil War–era dwellings housed U.S. officers stationed in the Presidio. Pershing Hall is in the background.

➤Turn left onto Moraga and walk to Funston Avenue. You will pass Pershing Square on your left. The square commemorates Brigadier General John Joseph Pershing's wife and three children who perished in a house fire on this site in 1915 while Pershing was on military duty on the Mexican border. General Pershing would go on to command the American expeditionary force in Europe during World War I. Just beyond the square, at the corner of Graham Street, stands the Spanish-style one-story building that served as the Presidio's Officers Club. A bit farther on is the post chapel, built in 1864 but modified in the 1950s.

➤At the corner of Moraga and Funston Avenue, turn right and walk around to the back of Pershing Hall and the corner of Funston and Hardee Street. An unmarked trail leads up the hill behind Pershing Hall.

➤Pass to the right of the gate just ahead and walk uphill on the asphalt path—which after about 30 feet turns into an uneven dirt surface. You are now entering the Presidio forest planted by the Army during the 1880s.

➤The trail soon forks into three paths. Take the path to the left. This broad path runs level for about 60 feet, after which it descends gently past lush undergrowth. Depending on the time of year, you may encounter people picking wild blackberries along this stretch.

➤Continue on the broad main path as it climbs, passing on your left a metal gate where a short drive leads up toward the main path. Notice how the light filters down through the forest's dense overstory.

During the course of this walk, you will pass several trails that meet the main trail from the left. Ignore these side trails—which are not marked on the map—and stay on the main trail.

➤As the trail continues to climb, you will pass a marker for a habitat restoration area. This project is designed to protect certain endangered species, among them Presidio clarkia, Marin dwarf flax, San Francisco owl's clover, coast rock cress, and the San Francisco gum plant. Please stay on the trail to avoid disturbing these fragile plants.

➤The trail curves to the left and passes by redwood trees in the midst of a cypress grove.

➤As the trail comes out into the open and levels out, it parallels a wire-and-post fence delineating another habitat restoration area on your right.

➤Follow the trail as it passes by a beautiful open meadow off to your right. To your right, at the top of the meadow, you can spot the guardrail along Arguello Boulevard.

➤The trail continues out in the open, with gentle ups and downs, and parallels Arguello Boulevard at a distance.

The trail passes through a striking stand of Monterey pines. These trees have lost all their lower branches, and their foliage starts quite high on their trunks. On your right, the post-and-cable fence marking the sensitive habitat area continues to run alongside the trail. Take a moment to stop, look back at the dips and curves of the trail, and try to remember that you are actually in the midst of a densely populated city.

➤About 50 feet beyond the stand of Monterey pines, you will reach a prominent trail juncture which is marked on the map. Do not take the left-hand trail that descends steeply into the shaded forest. Follow the right-hand path that leads up the hill. This trail climbs steeply and then levels out in a series of gentle ups and downs.

➤About 150 feet beyond the last trail juncture, a second post-and-cable fence starts up, this time on your left. Directly across on your right is a narrow path that leads up to Inspiration Point with its overlook and parking lot.

➤Turn right onto the narrow path to Inspiration Point and walk uphill about 100 feet to the overlook. Here you will find a great view of the Presidio's forest and a glimpse of the bay beyond. A historical marker at the overlook shows photographs taken from this ridge in 1880, when the dunes were bare between here and the Main Post, and in 1882, after the Army had planted thousands of trees in orderly rows.

➤Retrace your steps back to the main trail and turn right.

➤The trail dips up and down gently as it curves around the hillside below Inspiration Point and passes another sensitive habitat area on your left.

➤Farther on, a wide path—which is marked on the map—crosses the main trail. It leads up to the right to a gate near

of interest

Restoring the Habitats of Endangered Species

As you walk through the Presidio, the Marin Headlands, and other parts of the Golden Gate National Recreation Area, you may come upon signs announcing that you have just passed an "Endangered Species Habitat Restoration" area. What are these areas, and why are they so important?

Many of the plants commonly seen in the Bay Area are not native to the region. Even the eucalyptus, Monterey pine, and Monterey cypress trees that seem so much at home here were introduced to help break the winds that hammer these exposed headlands and clifftops. Since the National Park Service took over these areas from the U.S. Army and other landowners in recent years, it has made habitat restoration—especially for endangered species—a top priority.

Often this means removing introduced plants that have altered local ecosystems significantly enough to make them inhospitable to endangered species like the mission blue butterfly in the Marin Headlands or rare native plants like coast rock cress or San Francisco gum plant in the Presidio. In the case of the mission blue, Monterey pines prevent the healthy survival of the butterfly's host plant, the silver lupine.

These restoration projects do not mean that the park service will remove all the trees and other nonnative plants in the GGNRA. In fact, it is committed to preserving the historic forests planted here by the military and early settlers. At the same time, however, where it makes good environmental sense, park employees and volunteers will continue to remove introduced species, allowing native plants—and in some cases, insects, birds, and animals—to reclaim their home turf.

Please aid in this effort by always staying on clearly marked trails and heeding the signs that herald the return of native species. For more information, contact any GGNRA visitor center.

Arguello Boulevard and the parking area for the Presidio Golf Course. Ignore this cross trail and continue straight ahead on the main trail.

➤You will pass through a eucalyptus grove, and beyond it, you will begin to see the homes that line West Pacific Avenue.

➤The path leads to a small gate that sits along West Pacific. Walk around this gate, and turn left onto the narrow path that parallels West Pacific.

➤Follow this path as it broadens and descends toward the tennis courts of the Julius Kahn Playground. The path, running a straight course along West Pacific for about one-half mile, passes through a grove of Monterey cypress. These expressive trees, their branches outspread, look like a group of dancers poised and waiting for the music to begin.

➤Follow the trail as it passes to the right of Julius Kahn Playground, with its children's play area, restrooms, and softball diamond. Notice the elegant homes off to your right along West Pacific Avenue.

➤Just after passing the softball diamond, the path heads into a dark tunnel of trees. In this cypress grove—this mysterious and enchanted forest—branches grope up toward the light and interweave to create a canopy so tangled and dense that it could keep you dry during a mild rain shower.

➤Stay on the trail that parallels the low wall on the Presidio's perimeter. Ignore the paths that lead off to the left. Soon you will be able to see cars entering the Presidio through the Presidio Gate up ahead.

➤Walk uphill along the path and then to the left of the curving roadway—West Pacific Avenue—for a few paces until you reach a crosswalk.

The crosswalk marks West Pacific's intersection with the Lovers' Lane Trail. Immediately recognizable by its straight, steep descent lined with lampposts, Lovers' Lane is the oldest trail in San Francisco. The Spanish used it to travel between the Presidio and Mission Dolores 3 miles away. Later it became the trail by which off-duty officers would leave the Presidio to visit civilian San Francisco—and often their sweethearts, hence its current name.

➤Turn left onto Lovers' Lane and descend past the group of brick houses built in the 1930s. Imagine Presidio life during its heyday, when these substantial homes housed the lively families of enlisted men.

➤At the bottom of the hill, cross MacArthur Avenue, continue over a small brick footbridge, and then climb for a short block to the intersection where Barnard Avenue dead-ends into Presidio Boulevard as Presidio makes a 90-degree turn.

➤Cross Presidio at the crosswalk and continue straight ahead for 1 block along Presidio to Funston Avenue. Four large homes flank this block of Presidio. These fine examples of Queen Anne and Stick-style architecture were built in the 1880s as residences for officers.

➤Cross Funston and turn left. At this point—where Presidio intersects Funston—you are passing the original entrance to the Spanish-era Presidio.

➤Walk uphill on Funston for 1 block along "Officers' Row." Built in 1862, these homes are the oldest still standing in the Presidio. The simple, three- or four-bedroom wooden houses were built to house officers who until then had shared six rooms in an adobe building left by the Spanish.

➤Turn right at Moraga and walk 5 blocks to Montgomery.

➤Turn right onto Montgomery and walk 3.5 blocks to the Visitor Information Center and the end of this walk.

walk 17

Marin Headlands: Wolf Ridge Loop

General location: On the Marin Headlands, directly across the Golden Gate Bridge from San Francisco.

Special attractions: Historical landmarks; beach; spectacular views of San Francisco, Marin Headlands, and ocean.

Difficulty rating: Difficult, with some long uphill stretches. The trail surface is often uneven.

Distance: 5.5 miles.

Estimated time: 3 hours.

Services: Restrooms, visitor information center.

Restrictions: Not wheelchair accessible. Please note that the Pacific Coast Trail portion of this walk is subject to continual erosion and the National Park Service reroutes the trail as necessary. Watch for clearly marked detours. There is little shade on this trail; we recommend that you bring a hat and water bottle. Be careful on cliffs and at the beach; stay on the trails and heed the signs warning that "people have been swept away from the rocks and drowned." Each year, the park service rescues numerous people—and dogs—who fall off cliffs or get swept away by heavy surf or riptides. Dogs must either be leashed or under voice control, depending on where you are walking in the Golden Gate National Recreation Area (GGNRA). In some areas, pets are even prohibited entirely to protect sensitive resources. Dog droppings must be picked up. Contact the GGNRA headquarters at Fort Mason for a listing of pet regulations.

For more information: Contact GGNRA headquarters at Fort Mason or the Marin Headlands Visitor Center.

Getting started: This walk begins in the parking lot at the far end of Fort Cronkhite in the Marin Headlands.

(1) For freeway exits into San Francisco from the East Bay or the San Francisco Peninsula, refer to "Meet San Francisco" earlier in this book. From the intersection of Market, Ninth, Hayes, and Larkin Streets near the Civic Center, veer left onto Hayes and go 3 blocks. Turn right onto Franklin Street and go approximately 1.75 miles to Lombard Street. Turn left onto Lombard and continue 3 miles, following the signs to the Golden Gate Bridge. Immediately after crossing the bridge, take the Alexander Avenue exit. Turn left at the first stop, go under the freeway, and then turn right onto Conzelman Road, following the signs for the Golden Gate National Recreation Area and Marin Headlands. After climbing steeply into the headlands for 1.5 miles—the views are spectacular—turn right onto Mc-Cullough Road and head downhill, away from the ocean. Turn left onto Bunker Road, drive past Field Road, which

Wolf Ridge Loop and Rodeo Lagoon

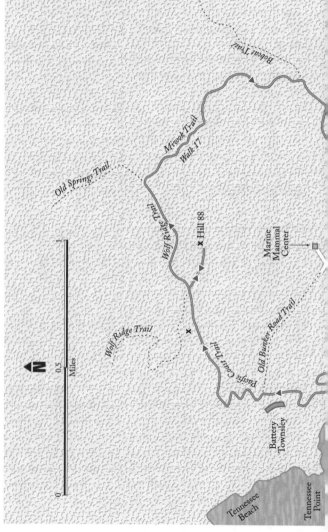

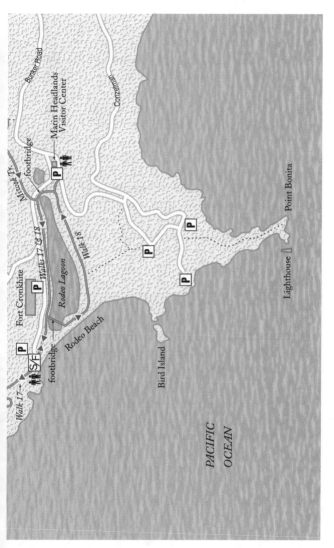

leads to the Marin Headlands Visitor Center, and continue past Rodeo Lagoon and the buildings of Fort Cronkhite. Drive to the end of the road and park in the parking lot.

Note: Coming from the San Francisco Peninsula, you can avoid downtown San Francisco by taking Interstate 280 North to the 19th Avenue/Park Presidio exit just beyond Daly City. Continue on California Highway 1 North—over Junipero Serra Boulevard, 19th Avenue, and Park Presidio—to the Golden Gate Bridge.

(2) From Marin County, drive on U.S. Highway 101 South and take the Sausalito exit just before the Golden Gate Bridge. Then turn left at the first stop and go under the freeway. Turn right onto Conzelman Road, following the signs for the Golden Gate National Recreation Area and Marin Headlands. After climbing steeply into the headlands 1.5 miles—the views are spectacular—turn right onto McCullough Road and head downhill, away from the ocean. Turn left onto Bunker Road, drive past Field Road, which leads to the Marin Headlands Visitor Center, and continue past Rodeo Lagoon and the buildings of Fort Cronkhite. Drive to the end of the road and park in the parking lot.

Public transportation: Bus 76 of the San Francisco Municipal Railway (Muni) runs to Fort Cronkhite only on Sundays and some holidays. It is wheelchair accessible. Contact Muni for information about schedules, fares, and accessibility.

Overview: Situated directly north of San Francisco, just off the Golden Gate Bridge, the Marin Headlands represent a resource rich in human history and natural beauty. This vigorous walk takes you deep into the headlands, where you will discover remnants of the area's military past, breathtaking vistas, and a landscape both wild and accessible. It is quite a hike, climbing 880 feet from sea level and then dropping back down to the ocean. The walk links four separate trails to make a pleasing loop: the Pacific Coast Trail, the Wolf Ridge Trail, the Miwok Trail, and a portion of the Rodeo Lagoon Loop (see Walk 18) that runs alongside Bunker Road.

This walk begins at Fort Cronkhite, one of the many U.S. Army facilities in the Bay Area turned over to the National Park Service in recent years. Here you will find a picnic area—the grills are wheelchair accessible—restrooms, and water. Public showers serve the handful of surfers hardy enough to risk the savage undertows that make the surf here not altogether safe.

The rolling coastal hills and dramatic seaside cliffs of the headlands have been home to Army gun emplacements since the mid-19th century, and it was only with the introduction of long-range missiles that the batteries here were no longer needed. As you climb ever higher into the headlands, watch for the ruins of these batteries. For more information about the emplacements, ask at the Marin Headlands Visitor Center. See "Getting started" above for directions to the visitor center; Walk 18 also takes you there.

Although the military and local ranchers have altered this landscape—blasting into hillsides and allowing cattle to decimate native grasses—the headlands remain a rich habitat for many varieties of plants and animals, especially birds. The distinctive coastal scrub, made up of a mix of such plants as California sagebrush, California blackberry, coyote bush, sticky monkeyflower, currant, and the ubiquitous poison oak, covers these hillsides. Common wildflowers include California poppies, Douglas iris, blue dicks, rock cress, lupines, and columbine. You will almost certainly see small lizards darting across the trail, and lucky walkers may catch a glimpse of deer, foxes, and bobcats. Birds frequently seen in the headlands include western grebes, cormorants, herons, turkey vultures, gulls, great horned owls, scrub jays,

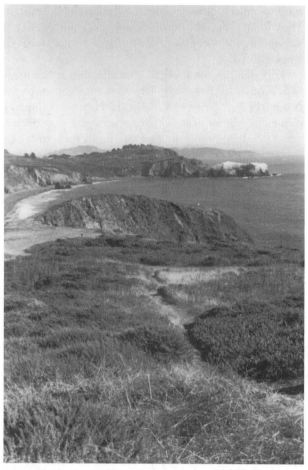

The Marin Headlands offer some of the most spectacular vistas in the Bay Area.

and even the endangered brown pelican. Ask at the visitor center about Hawk Hill, also known as Hill 129, stopping place in the early fall for thousands of migrating raptors.

As you climb into the headlands, do not forget to look behind you, back to the lovely curve of Rodeo Beach and, across the water, to the Golden Gate Bridge and the city of San Francisco, luminous in sunlight or shrouded in fog.

Note: This walk can be combined with Walk 18, Marin Headlands: Rodeo Lagoon. At the end of this walk, instead of turning right along Bunker Road, turn left and walk to the guard rail alongside Bunker Road. Descend the short set of stairs, and follow Walk 18 in reverse as it passes by the Marin Headlands Visitor Center and the southern edge of the lagoon, emerging on Rodeo Beach within view of the parking lot and the start of this walk.

The walk

➤Start at the western end of the parking lot at Fort Cronkhite. Facing the beach, exit the parking lot and turn right. Pass through a gate and onto the old asphalt road—marked "Pacific Coast Trail"—that leads up into the hills.

The Wolf Ridge Loop is made up of three separate trails—the Pacific Coast Trail, the Wolf Ridge Trail, and the Miwok Trail—plus a piece of the Rodeo Lagoon Loop.

You will discover that sections of the paved Pacific Coast Trail have slumped and are slowly sliding down the hillsides. Watch for clearly marked detours.

➤Follow the trail as it curves slightly to the right, and note the concrete fortifications—gun batteries—on the hillsides above.

As you switchback into the headlands, you can look back and see increasingly spectacular views of Fort Cronkhite,

Rodeo Beach, the Pacific, and the city of San Francisco itself. Among the San Francisco sights you can catch on clearer days are Sutro Tower and Twin Peaks, the forested hills of Lands End, and the sandy expanse of Ocean Beach.

Listen for the bleating of the foghorns and the banging of the buoy bells as you climb higher into these coastal hills so typical of Northern California.

➤You will circle behind Battery Townsley and see the battered steel doors barring entry into the vegetation-covered concrete structure. "Battery Townsley" and the date 1938 are painted above the doors.

➤As you leave the battery, you will head into the heart of the headlands, leaving the ocean behind. The trail descends here, before climbing once again. Just where it begins its upward climb, the main trail meets another trail, called Old Bunker Road Trail, coming in from the right. This trail, which you do not want to take, originates near the Marine Mammal Center just above Fort Cronkhite.

➤Continue to follow the Pacific Coast Trail, which curves to the left.

Very near the top of the ridge, the trail levels out and even begins to descend. At your left, you will see another gun emplacement.

➤Farther on, follow the trail as it joins a paved road. At first relatively flat, the road begins to climb steeply again, toward the top of Hill 88. Watch for small lizards skittering across the asphalt.

➤You will come to a junction on the roadway, with a sign off to your left that indicates that you should turn left off the roadway and then immediately right to join the Wolf Ridge Trail. The sign also indicates the location of the Pacific Coast Trail and Tennessee Valley. You are now 2.3 miles from Rodeo Beach.

➤Ultimately you will take the Wolf Ridge Trail, but before doing so, continue up the roadway to the top of Hill 88, where you will find the ruins of a military radar station built during the early 1950s. This "ghost" station is a wonderful spot for a picnic lunch and offers some of the best views on this walk.

➤Retrace your steps down the roadway to the turnoff for Wolf Ridge Trail. Turn right and begin descending the dirt Wolf Ridge Trail, which circles around the back side of Hill 88.

➤Wolf Ridge Trail descends steeply, carrying you into the cooler, more moist microclimate—complete with denser vegetation—on the shady back side of Hill 88. Because it is so steep, it is easy to get going too fast on this dusty trail. Watch your footing.

You may see a variety of birds—from finches to hawks—together with snakes, more lizards, and even an occasional bobcat or black-tailed deer. Off to the left you can see the Tennessee Valley Trail and, farther off, the houses of Mill Valley scattered among the trees. Butterflies flutter from bush to bush.

➤After the steep descent, the trail levels out and even climbs a bit, before a final descent into a fenced turnaround. Off to your left you will spot a locked gate and a sign that reads, "Habitat Area. Closed for Habitat Restoration." The trail curves right onto a dirt road. This is the Miwok Trail.

➤Descend the Miwok Trail. Mountain bikers often climb this long, steep road, but there is plenty of room for both walkers and bikers. If you are keen eyed, you may see the lodge of a dusky-footed woodrat. You will see tall stalks of fennel and thick thickets of thistle.

➤On your left as you descend, please note the habitat restoration project under way. Park volunteers have placed landscaping fabric over the plants currently choking the hillside, to "assist in the recovery of native plant species." To help further this project, please do not step off the trail.

►Soon you will see ahead the main highway—Bunker Road—leading into Fort Cronkhite and, off to your left, the buildings of the public stables. Stay to the right on the trail; do not go left onto the Bobcat Trail. The Miwok Trail passes by a marshy area on your left and ends beside an old warehouse on Bunker Road. Straight across the road lie the vivid green waters of Rodeo Lagoon.

►Cross Bunker Road and, turning right, walk on the trail alongside the lagoon. This trail will take you back to Fort Cronkhite and the end of this walk.

walk 18

Marin Headlands: Rodeo Lagoon

(See map on pages 208 and 209)

  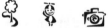

General location: On the Marin Headlands, directly across the Golden Gate Bridge from San Francisco.

Special attractions: Waterfowl; beach; Marine Mammal Center; views of San Francisco, Marin Headlands, ocean, and bay.

Difficulty rating: Easy, except for brief stretch walking in deep sand on beach.

Distance: 1.25 miles.

Estimated time: 45 minutes.

Services: Restrooms, visitor information center.

Restrictions: Not wheelchair accessible. Be careful on cliffs or at the beach; heed signs on Rodeo Beach warning of dangerous cliffs and surf. Each year, the National Park Service rescues numerous people—and dogs—who fall off cliffs or get swept away by heavy surf or riptides. Dogs must either be leashed or under voice control, depending on where you are walking in the Golden Gate National Recreation Area (GGNRA). In some areas, pets are even prohibited entirely to protect sensitive resources. Dog droppings must be picked up. Contact the GGNRA headquarters at Fort Mason for a listing of pet regulations. Mountain bikes are not allowed on this trail; they are allowed elsewhere in the Marin Headlands. The waters of Rodeo Lagoon are contaminated. Do not drink them or swim in them. Fishing and boating are also forbidden in the lagoon. Heed the signs on Rodeo Beach warning of "dangerous cliffs and surf."

For more information: Contact GGNRA headquarters at Fort Mason or the Marin Headlands Visitor Center.

Getting started: This walk begins in the parking lot at the far end of Fort Cronkhite in the Marin Headlands.

(1) For freeway exits into San Francisco from the East Bay or the San Francisco Peninsula, refer to "Meet San Francisco" earlier in this book. From the intersection of Market, Ninth, Hayes, and Larkin Streets near the Civic Center, veer left onto Hayes and go 3 blocks. Turn right onto Franklin Street and go approximately 1.75 miles to Lombard Street. Turn left onto Lombard and continue 3 miles, following the signs to the Golden Gate Bridge. Immediately after crossing the bridge, take the Alexander Avenue exit. Turn left at the first stop, go under the freeway, and then turn right onto Conzelman Road, following the signs for the Golden Gate National Recreation Area and Marin Headlands. After climbing steeply into the headlands for 1.5 miles—the views are spectacular—turn right onto McCullough Road and head downhill, away from the ocean. Turn left onto Bunker Road, drive past Field Road, which

leads to the Marin Headlands Visitor Center, and continue past Rodeo Lagoon and the buildings of Fort Cronkhite. Drive to the end of the road and park in the parking lot.

Note: Coming from the San Francisco Peninsula, you can avoid downtown San Francisco by taking Interstate 280 North to the 19th Avenue/Park Presidio exit just beyond Daly City. Continue on California Highway 1 North—over Junipero Serra Boulevard, 19th Avenue, and Park Presidio—to the Golden Gate Bridge.

(2) From Marin County, drive on U.S. Highway 101 South and take the Sausalito exit just before the Golden Gate Bridge. Then turn left at the first stop and go under the freeway. Turn right onto Conzelman Road, following the signs for the Golden Gate National Recreation Area and Marin Headlands. After climbing steeply into the headlands 1.5 miles—the views are spectacular—turn right onto McCullough Road and head downhill, away from the ocean. Turn left onto Bunker Road, drive past Field Road, which leads to the Marin Headlands Visitor Center, and continue past Rodeo Lagoon and the buildings of Fort Cronkhite. Drive to the end of the road and park in the parking lot.

Public transportation: Bus 76 of the San Francisco Municipal Railway (Muni) runs to Fort Cronkhite only on Sundays and some holidays. It is wheelchair accessible. Contact Muni for information about schedules, fares, and accessibility.

Overview: The Rodeo Lagoon loop is among the shortest walks in this guide, but it offers many pleasures, especially to those who love watching birds. Be sure to bring your binoculars and your camera. This walk is ideal for families with kids, because of its brevity, lack of challenging hills, and proximity to the beach.

Rodeo Beach, where this walk begins, is a marvelous place to walk in the sand and enjoy a picnic or a little sunbathing, weather permitting. Rodeo Lagoon lies adjacent to the beach. In winter, powerful waves cross the beach and enter the lagoon. This annual infusion of salt water makes the lagoon an ideal habitat for certain plants and animals. As the ocean subsides with the arrival of spring, it leaves behind enough sand to reestablish the beach, separating lagoon from ocean once again.

Though the lagoon's waters are stagnant through much of the year, they provide rich nutrients for tiny aquatic animals and plants, which in turn attract all manner of hungry waterfowl—from snowy egrets to many varieties of ducks to the rare brown pelican. These pelicans, officially endangered, can be found on the lagoon during spring, summer, and fall. Salamanders mate here, and you can sometimes see raccoons, foxes, and other mammals in the dense brush along the shore.

Take your time as you circle Rodeo Lagoon. Perhaps you will encounter a local birdwatcher who will share with you—as one did with us—her deep knowledge of the birds that make their homes on these intensely green waters. This brief but lovely walk also leads you to the Marin Headlands Visitor Center, where the extremely helpful staff can answer almost any question about the headlands ecosystem. A special note for bird lovers: Ask at the visitor center about Hawk Hill, also known as Hill 129, stopping place in the early fall for thousands of migrating raptors.

Note: This walk may be combined with Walk 17, Marin Headlands: Wolf Ridge Loop. Walk 18 ends in the Fort Cronkhite parking lot, which is also the starting point for Walk 17. After doing the Rodeo Lagoon walk—and perhaps now armed with information from the visitor center—begin Walk 17 in the Fort Cronkhite parking lot.

The walk

➤Start in the parking lot at the far end of Fort Cronkhite. Facing the beach, exit the parking lot, cross Bunker Road, and turn left. Walk on the path alongside the roadway until you are opposite a wooden footbridge. This bridge leads to Rodeo Beach and the trail around Rodeo Lagoon.

At the bridge, interpretive panels describe the wildlife of the lagoon and the natural forces that shape the lagoon and beach each year.

➤Cross the bridge and turn left, walking in the deep sand of the beach at the edge of the lagoon.

You are almost certain to see waterfowl in the waters of the lagoon. On each of our visits, we saw snowy egrets, brown pelicans, and several varieties of ducks and gulls. Another

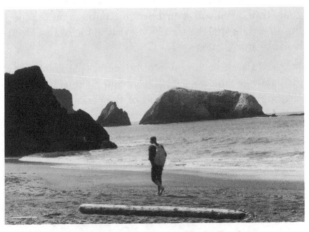

A beachcomber walks the sandy expanse of Rodeo Beach.

visitor was delighted to encounter green-backed herons, less commonly seen than great blue herons.

➤When you reach the opposite shore of the lagoon, turn left onto the clearly marked trail that leads away from the beach and up onto the hillside above the lagoon. At first the trail is quite sandy, making walking a little difficult, but the footing grows more stable as the path climbs.

Listen for the distinctive sound of the brown pelicans flapping their wings, and for the cries of the seals and sea lions in residence at the Marine Mammal Center across the lagoon.

➤As the trail begins to descend, it takes you through willow thickets and then into a veritable willow glade, so dense you can scarcely see the sky.

➤Soon after the trail comes back into the open and begins to climb again, note the sign off to your left reading "Lagoon Trail." You will return here to continue on the loop. But first walk straight ahead for a visit to the Marin Headlands Visitor Center.

➤Pass through a gate and into the center's parking lot. Immediately beyond the gate and to your right, you will find restrooms. Walk to the far end of the parking lot and the visitor center, which is housed in a historic white church.

The center features an excellent bookstore, interpretive displays, and a friendly and helpful staff—as do all the visitor centers in the Golden Gate National Recreation Area.

➤Upon exiting the visitor center, retrace your steps along the parking lot, through the gate, and back to the sign marking the continuation of the Lagoon Trail. Turn right.

➤Descend some wooden steps, and then as the trail levels out, cross a little wooden bridge.

The Marine Mammal Center

The Marine Mammal Center, just up the hill from Fort Cronkhite in the Marin Headlands, is a wonderful place—and it is open to visitors. Its mission is to "recognize our interdependence with marine mammals and our responsibility to use our awareness, compassion, and intelligence to ensure their survival and the conservation of their habitat."

In pursuit of that mission, the center each year treats nearly 1,000 ill and injured marine mammals in its hospital. Its education programs—which may involve slide shows, artifacts, or excursions along the coast—reach many thousands of people, helping them better understand the whales, dolphins, otters, seals, and sea lions the center serves. And the center's important science program conducts studies of the threats—both from disease and environmental changes—that these marine mammals face.

As a nonprofit organization, the Marine Mammal Center depends upon memberships, donations, and volunteers to achieve its mission. If you would like to help, contact the center.

➤Climb a short set of stairs that takes you up to the guardrail alongside Bunker Road.

➤Turn left, and follow the dirt trail alongside the lagoon, back to Fort Cronkhite and the end of this walk. As you head back toward the ocean, you will again have great views of the many birds—some perched on old pilings—that spend time on the nutrient-rich waters of Rodeo Lagoon.

Appendix A: Other Sights

San Francisco and the surrounding region offer an almost infinite array of attractions. Those listed below are just a sampling of the many to be enjoyed in the greater Bay Area. Not all involve walking, but each has delighted millions of tourists and residents. Have a great time.

In San Francisco

Cable Car Barn and Museum
1201 Mason Street
415-474-1887

This wonderful museum—set in the still-operating cable car powerhouse or winding house—takes you through the history of San Francisco's legendary cable car system. Its excellent exhibits are well worth the visit, but it is the viewing area downstairs—where you can watch the great wheels wind the cables—that truly fascinates most visitors.

San Francisco Zoo
Sloat Boulevard and 45th Avenue
415-753-7080
www.sfzoo.com

The San Francisco Zoo features the Doegler Primate Discovery Center, where you can watch apes and monkeys in environments that simulate their natural habitats. More than 1,000 species make their home at the zoo, including Australian koalas, seldom seen in this country. Interactive and computer exhibits are among the educational attractions, as is a mini-zoo designed specifically for kids.

Mission Dolores
Dolores and 16th Streets
415-621-8203

San Francisco's oldest structure—it was built in 1782—Mission Dolores is a monument to this city's Spanish founders and to the influence of Catholic missions in early California. After surviving several major earthquakes, the 1906 fire, and two centuries of use, this modest mission remains an important part of the Mission District, to which it lends its name.

Outside San Francisco

Alcatraz Island
San Francisco Bay
415-705-1042 or 415-556-0560
www.nps.gov/alcatraz

Home for many years to a famed federal prison, this island is one of the most frequently visited places in the Golden Gate National Recreation Area. Besides touring the cellhouse, you can visit the first lighthouse on the West Coast; walk along the island's cliffs for heartstopping views of San Francisco, the bay, and passing ships; and learn more about the natural history of this austere and intriguing place. To reach Alcatraz from San Francisco, take a Blue & Gold ferry from Pier 41. Blue & Gold ferries from Pier 41 will also take you to Angel Island, used during World War II as a Japanese internment center and now a state park (www.angelisland.org).

Bay Area Discovery Museum
East Fort Baker
557 McReynolds Road, Sausalito 94965
415-331-2129
www.badm.org

This kid-oriented museum—for ages 1 through 10—teaches with hands-on exhibits about the Bay Area's rich human and natural history. It is a perfect place to spend an afternoon with the family. While at East Fort Baker, you can also check out the fishing pier and abandoned gun batteries, take a pleasant walk to Sausalito Point, or just enjoy the sunny weather on this side of the bay.

Muir Woods National Monument

Mill Valley, CA 94941

415-388-2595

www.nps.gov/muwo

Named for John Muir, the father of modern conservation, Marin County's Muir Woods preserves a grand remnant of the virgin redwood forests that once flourished through much of the Bay Area. The hiking trails in Muir Woods range from an easy 2 miles to a strenuous 8.5 miles. This extremely popular piece of the Golden Gate National Recreation Area is often very crowded on summer weekends.

Point Reyes National Seashore

Point Reyes Station, CA 94956-9799

415-663-1092

www.nps.gov/pore

For walkers who prefer a wilder experience than San Francisco can offer, this absolutely gorgeous oceanfront park 40 miles north of San Francisco features 32,000 acres of designated wilderness, with 70-some miles of trails and several campgrounds. At Point Reyes, you can also visit an 1860s dairy ranch, ascend to a historic lighthouse, and take an interpretive walk that explains the earthquakes that periodically rumble through this beautiful place.

The Wine Country

In the valleys of Napa, Sonoma, Mendocino, and Lake Counties north of San Francisco

This region, rich in wineries and great food, is a marvelous pleasure ground. Not only can you sip world-class vintages here, but you will want to tour the back roads, enjoy spectacular ocean views, walk in the redwoods, and spend delightful nights in some of the best bed-and-breakfasts anywhere. A great guide to this magical region is *The Insiders' Guide to California's Wine Country* by Phil Barber and Phyllis Zauner.

Appendix B: Contact Information

Throughout this book, we have recommended that you contact the local attractions, museums, and visitor centers we mention to confirm opening times, locations, and entrance fees. The list below gives you the addresses and phone numbers (as well as websites, where available) for the places we've mentioned.

The San Francisco Convention and Visitors Bureau has a wealth of information available about San Francisco and the Bay Area. Stop by the Visitor Information Center at Hallidie Plaza, or call the bureau's helpful staff.

San Francisco Convention and Visitors Bureau, Visitor Information Center, 900 Market Street, Hallidie Plaza (at Market and Powell Streets, next to the cable car turnaround), San Francisco 94102-2804; 415-391-2000; www.sfvisitor.org.

Send mail requests to:

San Francisco Convention and Visitors Bureau, Main Office, 201 Third Street, San Francisco 94103; 415-974-6900.

The following excellent San Francisco websites offer information on lodging, restaurants, and shopping: http://citysearch7.com; http://sanfrancisco.sidewalk.com.

Activities, Attractions, and Museums

Ansel Adams Center for Photography, 250 4th Street, San Francisco 94013; 415-495-7000.

Asian Art Museum of San Francisco, Music Concourse, Golden Gate Park, Tea Garden Drive, between John F. Kennedy and Martin Luther King, Jr. Drives, San Francisco 94111; 415-379-8801; www.asianart.org.

California Academy of Sciences (Steinhart Aquarium, Morrison Planetarium, and Natural History Museum), Music Concourse, Golden Gate Park, Concourse Drive, between John F. Kennedy and Martin Luther King, Jr. Drives, San Francisco 94111; 415-750-7145; www.calacademy.org.

California Historical Society, 678 Mission Street, San Francisco 94105; 415-357-1848; www.calhist.org.

California Palace of the Legion of Honor, Lincoln Park (34th Avenue and Clement Street), San Francisco 94121; 415-863-3330; www.famsf.org.

The Cannery, 2801 Leavenworth Street, San Francisco 94133; 415-771-3112.

Center for the Arts at Yerba Buena Gardens, 701 Mission Street, San Francisco 94103; 415-978-2787; www.yerbabuenaarts.org.

Chinese Culture Center, Holiday Inn, 3rd floor, 750 Kearny Street, San Francisco 94108; 415-986-1822; www.c-c-c.org.

Chinese Historical Society of America Museum, 644 Broadway, Suite 402, San Francisco 94111; 415-391-1188.

City Lights Books, 261 Columbus Avenue, San Francisco 94133; 415-362-8193.

Coit Tower, Telegraph Hill Boulevard south of Lombard Street, San Francisco 94133; 415-362-0808.

Embarcadero Center, Main office: 415-772-0500, Information hotline: 800-733-6318.

The Exploratorium, Palace of Fine Arts, 3601 Lyon Street, San Francisco 94123; 415-361-0360; www.exploratorium.edu.

Galeria de la Raza/Studio 24, 2857 24th Street, San Francisco 94110; 415-826-8009.

Ghirardelli Square, 900 North Point Street, San Francisco 94109; 415-775-5500.

Gulf of the Farallones National Marine Sanctuary Visitor Center, Old Coast Guard Station, Golden Gate Promenade; 415-561-6622.

Haas-Lilienthal House, 2007 Franklin Street, San Francisco 94109; 415-441-3000.

Marine Mammal Center, off Bunker Road, Sausalito 94965; 415-289-7325; www.tmmc.org.

The Mexican Museum, Fort Mason Center, Building D, Laguna Street and Marina Boulevard, San Francisco 94133; 415-441-0445; 415-441-0404 (recorded information).

M. H. de Young Memorial Museum, Music Concourse, Golden Gate Park, Tea Garden Drive, between John F. Kennedy and Martin Luther King, Jr. Drives, San Francisco 94111; 415-863-3330; www.famsf.org.

Musée Mecanique, Cliff House, 1090 Point Lobos Avenue, San Francisco 94121; 415-386-1170.

Museo ItaloAmericano, Fort Mason Center, Laguna Street and Marina Boulevard, San Francisco 94133; 415-673-2200; www.well.com/user/museo.

The Museum of the City of San Francisco, The Cannery, 3rd floor, 2801 Leavenworth Street, San Francisco 94133; 415-928-0289; www.sfmuseum.org.

National Japanese American Historical Society, 1840 Sutter Street, San Francisco 94115; 415-776-0661.

North Beach Museum, 1435 Stockton Street, San Francisco 94133; 415-626-7070.

The Octagon House, 2645 Gough Street, San Francisco 94123; 415-441-7512.

USS *Pampanito*, Pier 45, Fisherman's Wharf, San Francisco 94133; 415-929-0202; www.maritime.org/pamphome.shtml.

PIER 39, Fisherman's Wharf, San Francisco 94133; 415-981-7437.

Precita Eyes Mural Arts and Visitor Center, 2981 24th Street, San Francisco 94110; 415-285-2287; www.precitaeyes.org.

San Francisco Art Institute, 800 Chestnut Street, San Francisco 94133; 415-771-7020; www.sfai.edu.

San Francisco Camera Obscura and Holograph Gallery, 1096 Point Lobos Avenue, San Francisco 94121; 415-750-0415.

San Francisco Craft and Folk Art Museum, Fort Mason Center, Building A, Marina Boulevard and Buchanan Street, San Francisco 94123; 415-775-0990; www.sfcraftandfolk.org.

San Francisco Museum of Modern Art, 151 Third Street, San Francisco 94103; 415-357-4000; www.sfmoma.org.

SkyDeck at Embarcadero Center, Deck 1, Embarcadero Center, San Francisco 94111; 415-772-0555; www.sfskydeck.com.

Public Beaches, Gardens, and Parks

Golden Gate National Recreation Area (GGNRA) Headquarters, Fort Mason, Building 201, San Francisco 94123; 415-556-0560; www.nps.gov/goga.

Cliff House, Visitor Information Center; 415-556-8642.

Fort Mason Center, Calendar of events: 415-441-3400; Recorded information: 415-979-3010.

Fort Point National Historic Site, Visitor Information Center; 415-556-1693.

Marin Headlands, Visitor Information Center; 415-331-1540.

Presidio of San Francisco, Visitor Information Center; 415-561-4323; 415-561-4314 TTY.

Golden Gate Park (GGP), McLaren Lodge, San Francisco 94117; 415-831-2700; http://civiccenter.ci.sf.ca.us/recpark/location.nsf.
In addition to the information desk at McLaren Lodge, there is a GGP Visitor Center at the Beach Chalet, 1000 Great Highway, on the western edge of the park. To receive information by mail, send $2.25 check (payable to San Francisco Recreation and Parks Department) to Golden Gate Park, Attention: Switchboard, Recreation and Parks Department, 501 Stanyan Street, San Francisco, CA 94117.

Japanese Tea Garden, 415-752-4227.

Strybing Arboretum and Botanical Gardens, 415-661-1316; www.strybing.org.

Other San Francisco City Parks

San Francisco Recreation and Parks Department,
McLaren Lodge, San Francisco 94117; 415-831-2700; http://civiccenter.ci.sf.ca.us/recpark/location.nsf.
The San Francisco Recreation and Parks Department oversees hundreds of parks, recreation centers, swimming pools, public works of art, and stairways.

San Francisco Maritime National Historical Park,
Aquatic Park to Hyde Street Pier, San Francisco
94109; 415-556-3002; www.nps.gov/safr.

Hyde Street Pier, foot of Hyde Street; San Francisco
94109; 415-556-3002.
Admission fee charged; open daily.

J. Porter Shaw Library, Building E, Fort Mason, San
Francisco 94133; 415-556-9870.
Call for hours.

San Francisco Maritime Museum, 900 Beach Street,
San Francisco 94109; 415-556-3002.
Admission free; open daily.

Public Golf Courses

Golden Gate Park Municipal Golf Course, Golden
Gate Park, San Francisco 94117; 415-751-8987.

Lincoln Park Municipal Golf Course, 34th Avenue and
Clement Street, San Francisco 94121; 415-221-9911.

Hotels

To find lodging that suits your tastes and pocketbook, call
the San Francisco Convention and Visitors Bureau official
reservation hotline at 1-888-782-9673 or 415-974-4499.
The bureau's list of 420 hotels, however, includes only those
enterprises that are bureau members. You might also want
to try San Francisco Visitors Hotel Hotline (listing more
than 300 hotels) at 1-800-511-5324 and San Francisco
Reservations at 1-800-677-1500. To identify the hotel you
want on the World Wide Web, try www.sfvisitor.org,
www.hotelres.com, or citysearch7.com.

Word of mouth is still one of the best ways to find a
great place to stay. Below we've listed a handful of excellent

hotels, including a few of the classic downtown hotels and several smaller "boutique" hostelries with plenty of character.

Beresford Hotel, 635 Sutter Street, San Francisco 94102; 415-673-9900.

Quaint European-flavored downtown hotel, featuring the White Horse Tavern.

The Clift Hotel, Geary and Taylor Streets, San Francisco 94102; 415-775-4700.

This satisfyingly old-fashioned and stately hotel, near Union Square, is steeped in tradition.

Fairmont Hotel, 950 Mason Street, San Francisco 94108; 415-772-5000.

An elegant, old San Francisco hotel—centrally located atop Nob Hill.

Grand Hyatt San Francisco Hotel, 345 Stockton Street, San Francisco 94108; 415-398-1234.

Just off Union Square, this modern hotel offers all the amenities.

Hotel Boheme, 444 Columbus Avenue, San Francisco 94133; 415-433-9111.

Travel & Leisure calls this small, beautifully appointed North Beach hotel the "hot address."

Hotel Rex, 652 Sutter Street, San Francisco 94102; 415-433-4434.

Not inexpensive, this small hotel features a literary theme, complete with rugged leather club chairs, antique writing desks, and quotes from San Francisco's favorite writers on the walls.

Hotel Sheehan, 620 Sutter Street, San Francisco 94102; 415-775-6500 or 1-800-848-1529.

Two blocks from Union Square, this European-style hotel features an indoor heated pool and 65 very moderately priced rooms.

Hotel Triton, 342 Grant Avenue, San Francisco 94108; 415-781-3566.

This postmodern fantasy sits at the heart of the city's French district. San Francisco artists assisted in the design of its unique guest rooms.

Hyatt Regency, 5 Embarcadero Center, San Francisco 94111; 415-788-1234.

Modern and centrally located near the Ferry Building, the Hyatt Regency is close to the waterfront, South of Market, and downtown. Known for its spectacular atrium lobby.

Mark Hopkins Intercontinental Hotel, 1 Nob Hill, San Francisco 94108; 415-392-3434.

Every visitor to San Francisco should visit the "Top of the Mark," the legendary cocktail lounge on the roof of this fashionable old hotel high on Nob Hill.

Renaissance Stanford Court Hotel, 905 California Street, San Francisco 94108; 415-989-3500.

A quiet and quality hotel just down Nob Hill from the Mark Hopkins.

San Remo Hotel, 2237 Mason Street, San Francisco 94133; 415-776-8688.

The best value for a European-style hotel in the city. This Italianate Victorian is close to Fisherman's Wharf and North Beach.

The Tuscan Inn, 425 North Point, San Francisco 94133; 415-561-1100.

Small and unpretentious, The Tuscan is a wonderful place to stay near Fisherman's Wharf.

Westin St. Francis Hotel, 335 Powell Street, San Francisco 94102; 415-397-7000.

Built in 1904, the St. Francis is a San Francisco landmark and the quintessential Union Square address.

Transportation

Amtrak, 510-238-4306 (for station information only), 800-872-7245 (for reservations and schedule information); www.amtrak.com.

AC Transit, Transbay Terminal, First and Mission Streets, San Francisco 94110; 415-817-1717 or 510-839-2931, 800-448-9790 TTY; www.actransit.dst.ca.us.

Bay Area Rail Transportation (BART), 800 Madison Street, Oakland 94607; 650-992-2278 (from San Francisco), 510-839-2220 TTY, 888-2-ELEVAT (station elevator information); www.bart.gov.

Bay Area Transit Information Project, www.transitinfo.org.
This website offers a comprehensive directory to San Francisco Bay Area transit services.

Blue & Gold Fleet, from PIER 39/Pier 41, Fisherman's Wharf, to Alameda/Oakland, Alcatraz, Angel Island, Sausalito, Tiburon, and Vallejo; 415-773-1188, 415-705-5555 (charge by phone); www.transitinfo.org/BlueGoldFleet.

Caltrain, 1250 San Carlos Avenue, San Carlos, CA 94070-1306; 800-660-4287, 650-508-6448 TTY; www.caltrain.com/caltrain.

Golden Gate Transit (GGT), Transbay Terminal, First and Mission Streets, San Francisco 94110; 415-923-2000 (from San Francisco), 415-455-2000 (from Marin County), 415-257-4554 TTY; www.goldengate.org.

Golden Gate Ferry, Golden Gate Ferry Terminal, Ferry Building, foot of Market Street, to Sausalito and Larkspur; 415-923-2000 (from San Francisco), 415-455-2000 (from Marin County), 415-257-4554 TTY; www.goldengate.org.

SamTrans, 415-817-1717 or 800-660-4287, 650-508-6448 TTY; www.caltrain.com/samtrans.

San Francisco Municipal Railway (Muni), 949 Presidio Avenue, San Francisco 94115; 415-673-MUNI or 415-817-1717, 415-923-6366 TTY; www.ci.sf.ca.us/muni.

TravInfo Bay Area Transit Service Information, 415-817-1717.

Appendix C: Great Tastes

San Francisco—together with the fertile countryside that surrounds it—is one of the great food places in America, and the city itself may be home to this country's greatest concentration of restaurants, something over 3,300. The following list includes just a few of the fine restaurants, cafés, and coffee houses to be found along the walks we've recommended, together with a few of our personal favorites. Anyone interested in surveying the full range of eateries to be found in the Bay Area should pick up one of the comprehensive restaurant guides to the region currently in print (see Appendix E).

Beach Chalet Brewery & Restaurant, 1000 Great Highway, San Francisco 94121; 415-386-8439.
Great casual food and beer brewed on the premises. Spectacular views of the ocean.

Betelnut, 2030 Union Street, San Francisco 94123; 415-929-8855.
Popular meeting place. Known for its delectable small and large plates of pan-Asian cuisine.

Buena Vista Café, 2765 Hyde Street, San Francisco 94133; 415-474-5044.
This landmark bar-café is the home of the original Irish coffee in America. Also famous for its breakfasts.

Café Bastille, 22 Belden Place, San Francisco 94104; 415-986-5673.
This classic, but casual French café with outside tables is right downtown.

Café Claude, 7 Claude Lane, San Francisco 94108; 415-392-3505.
A French find on a charming narrow street. Features wine, hors d'oeuvres, and daily specials. Jazz nightly.

Café De La Presse, 352 Grant Avenue, San Francisco 94108; 415-398-2680.

A bit of Paris with outdoor seating on a busy street. Great place to stop for coffee, a drink, or a copy of *Le Monde.*

Café deStijl, 1 Union Street, San Francisco 94111; 415-291-0808.

This elegantly industrial café near the Embarcadero is a tribute to Dutch modernist architecture. Great pie, and flamenco dinners on occasion.

Caffe Freddy's, 901 Columbus Avenue, San Francisco 94133; 415-922-0151.

This informal North Beach spot has imaginative sandwiches and light entrees. Great place to meet for coffee.

Caffe Greco, 423 Columbus Avenue, San Francisco 94133; 415-397-6261.

Outstanding among the many North Beach coffee houses. Our personal favorite.

Caffe Malvina, 1600 Stockton Street, San Francisco 94133; 415-391-1290.

Neighborhood hangout with great salads, gourmet pizza, and breakfasts all day long. Well-priced.

Caffe Museo, San Francisco Museum of Modern Art, 151 Third Street, San Francisco 94103; 415-357-4500.

This sleek indoor/outdoor café offers an appealing selection of light snacks and pastries.

Caffe Trieste, 601 Vallejo Street, San Francisco 94133; 415-392-6739.

Still the quintessential North Beach gathering spot for artists and writers.

Capp's Corner, 1600 Powell Street, San Francisco 94133; 415-989-2589.

Full and hearty Italian multi-course meals served family-style in a lively, old-time atmosphere.

Cliff House Restaurant, 1090 Point Lobos Avenue, San Francisco 94121; 415-386-3330; www.cliffhouse.com.
The greatest ocean views from every table. Upstairs is less formal than down. Excellent breakfasts.

Cooks and Company, Fort Mason Center, San Francisco 94123; 415-673-4137.
Situated at Fort Mason, Cooks and Company is a great place to pick up a quick snack or a lunch before setting out along the Marina Green.

Kuleto's, 221 Powell Street, San Francisco 94102; 415-397-7720.
This downtown standout sports a busy, sophisticated atmosphere and imaginative, delicious pasta. Reservations recommended.

DPD Restaurant, 901 Kearny Street, San Francisco 94133; 415-982-0471.
Simple and basic in atmosphere, DPD has been hailed as Chinatown's most interesting eating spot.

E&O Trading Company, 314 Sutter Street, San Francisco 94108; 415-693-0303.
"Pacific Rim" cuisine—among our favorite small plates are Indonesian corn fritters and lamb naan. Features a captivating interior upstairs, a brewery in the basement, and live music on the weekends.

Enrico's Sidewalk Café, 504 Broadway, San Francisco 94133; 415-982-6223.
Popular spot to see and be seen in North Beach. Terrace seating, music, lively atmosphere, and excellent food.

Firefly Restaurant, 4288 24th Street, San Francisco 94114; 415-821-7652.
This arty Noe Valley gathering place gets great reviews for its imaginative and subtle dishes.

Fog City Diner, 1300 Battery Street, San Francisco 94111; 415-982-2000.

This upscale diner near the Embarcadero and Levi's Plaza is best known for its crab cakes, oysters, and sand dabs.

Greens Restaurant, Fort Mason Center, Building A, San Francisco 94123; 415-771-6222.

Vegetarian cuisine par excellence. Spacious with gorgeous views of the bay.

The Helmand: Cuisine from Afghanistan, 430 Broadway, San Francisco 94133; 415-362-0641.

An oasis in the Broadway nightlife scene. Noted for its lamb dishes and spicy Afghani food.

Henry Chung's Original Hunan Restaurant, 924 Sansome Street, San Francisco 94133; 415-956-7727.

Hot and spicy cuisine from Hunan Province. High quality for many years. Great for large groups.

House of Nanking, 919 Kearny Street, San Francisco 94133; 415-421-1429.

This bare-bones storefront café at the edge of Chinatown is always crowded, but worth the wait. Great sizzling shrimp, always fresh ingredients, and inexpensive.

Il Fornaio Cucina Italiana, 1265 Battery Street, San Francisco 94111; 415-986-0100.

This casually elegant restaurant offers everything from pizza and pasta to full Italian meals.

Imperial Tea Court, 1411 Powell Street, San Francisco 94133; 415-788-6080.

Tea tasting for the true connoisseur of Chinese teas. Worth stopping in just for a look.

Julius' Castle, 1541 Montgomery Street, San Francisco 94133; 415-392-2222.

This pink stucco restaurant situated on the cliff below Coit

Tower is famous for its spectacular views of the bay and its pricey wine list.

Legion of Honor Café and Garden Terrace, California Palace of the Legion of Honor, Lincoln Park (34th Avenue and Clement Street), San Francisco 94121; 415-221-2233.

One of the finest museum cafés anywhere. Includes seating in a sculpture garden.

Liguria Bakery, 1700 Stockton Street, San Francisco 94133; 415-421-3786.

The Liguria sells only focaccia—the very best—made in its own ovens.

Mario's Bohemian Cigar Store Café, 566 Columbus Avenue, San Francisco 94133; 415-362-0536.

A landmark meeting place for North Beach locals. Try Mario's famous meatball sandwich.

Patisserie Delanghe, 1890 Fillmore Street, San Francisco 94115; 415-923-0711.

Classic, delicate French pastries.

Restaurant LuLu, 816 Folsom Street, San Francisco 94103; 415-495-5775.

South of Market not far from Yerba Buena Gardens. LuLu has a spectacular interior, extraordinary food, friendly service, and reasonable prices. Do not miss the rosemary chicken or mussels grilled over a wood fire.

Rose Pistola, 532 Columbus Avenue, San Francisco 94133; 415-399-0499.

One of San Francisco's hottest restaurants. Features innovative Northern Italian cuisine. Music after 9 P.M.

Swensen's Ice Cream, Union and Hyde, San Francisco 94109; 415-775-6818.

The original store of a well-known chain. The fabulous ice cream is made right here.

Tadich Grill, 240 California Street, San Francisco 94111; 415-391-1849.

Founded in 1849, this Financial District tradition is known for its seafood and the crowds it draws.

Tavolino Ristorante & Cicchetti Bar, 401 Columbus Avenue, San Francisco 94133; 415-392-1472.

This beautiful, light-filled North Beach restaurant features Venetian cuisine and friendly service.

Tosca Café, 242 Columbus Avenue, San Francisco 94133; 415-986-9651.

A North Beach joint famous for its long bar, film celebrity clientele, brandy-laced cappuccinos, and opera on the jukebox.

Vesuvio Café, 255 Columbus Avenue, San Francisco 94133; 415-362-3370.

More a bar than a café, Vesuvio's is a relic of the Beat era in North Beach. Go upstairs to the balcony for a bird's-eye view onto Columbus Avenue.

The Waterfront Restaurant & Café, Pier 7, San Francisco 94111; 415-398-7541.

Recently renovated, this beautiful restaurant sits right on the bay.

Yukol Place Thai Cuisine, 2380 Lombard Street, San Francisco 94123; 415-922-1599.

Great food, quiet atmosphere, and soothing on your wallet as well. Located 1 block off teeming Chestnut Street in the Marina District.

Yum Yum Fish, 2181 Irving Street, San Francisco 94122; 415-566-6433.

Located in the Sunset District near Golden Gate Park. There are a few tables, but Yum Yum sells most of its sushi and sashimi to go. Great stop on the way to a picnic in the park or at the beach.

Appendix D: Useful Phone Numbers

Please note that the area code for San Francisco is 415.

Police, Emergency 911, Non-emergency 553-0123, 626-4357 TTY.

San Francisco City & County Sheriff, Emergency 911, Information 650-364-1811 or 650-726-4435.

San Francisco Fire Department, Emergency 911 or 861-8020.

General Information and Referral, Northern California Council for the Community; 772-4357, 772-4440 TTY.

Hospitals, San Francisco General Hospital 206-8000, Emergency Department 206-8111, Emergency 206-8246 TTY, Health Information Services 206-8640.

National Park Police, San Francisco Field Office 556-5801.

Newspapers, *San Francisco Chronicle* (morning), 777-1111, *San Francisco Examiner* (evening), 777-2424.

Post Office, Rates and Information 284-0755.

Public Libraries, General Information 557-4400.

Road and Weather Conditions, 557-3755 or 800-427-7623.

State Highway Patrol, Emergency 911, Non-emergency accidents 707-648-5550, 707-648-5363 TTY.

Appendix E: Read All About It

One of the world's most desired destinations, San Francisco has been the subject of scores of guidebooks and travelogues, and as the West Coast's unrivaled literary center, the city on the bay has spawned countless novels, screenplays, and poems. The following bibliography is only a beginning. You will find many more books about this incredible city in its friendly bookstores, museum shops, and visitor centers. And remember that San Francisco has served as the setting for more than 100 feature films.

Fiction

Gina Berriault. *Women in Their Beds: New and Selected Stories.* Washington, DC: Counterpoint, 1997. A collection of 35 "jewel-box perfect" stories by an exceptional Bay Area writer.

Dashiell Hammett. *The Maltese Falcon.* New York: Vintage Crime/Black Lizard, 1992. Featuring Sam Spade, this atmospheric masterpiece of suspense fiction is set in the San Francisco of the 1920s.

Maxine Hong Kingston. *Tripmaster Monkey: His Fake Book.* New York: Vintage International, 1990. The story of a free-spirited Chinese-American writer in San Francisco during the late 1960s.

David Knowles. *The Secrets of the Camera Obscura.* San Francisco: Chronicle Books, 1994. A pulse-racing mystery that revolves around the Camera Obscura at the Cliff House next to Ocean Beach.

Armistead Maupin. *Tales of the City.* New York: Harper Perennial Library, 1994. Made into a miniseries for public television, this wise and funny novel—originally serialized in the *San Francisco Chronicle*—captures the magic and romance of Maupin's chosen city during the 1970s.

Frank Norris. *McTeague: A Story of San Francisco.* New York: New American Library, 1997. This gritty realist novel depicts San Francisco at the turn of the 20th century.

Amy Tan. *The Joy Luck Club.* New York: Ivy Books, 1994. A rich and involving novel set in San Francisco that recounts the interwoven stories of four Chinese immigrant mothers and their daughters.

Mark Twain. *Roughing It.* New York: New American Library, 1994. Partly fact and partly tall tale, this is Twain's colorful account of his early adulthood in Nevada, San Francisco (and elsewhere in California), and Hawaii.

Nonfiction

William Bronson. *The Earth Shook, the Sky Burned.* San Francisco: Chronicle Books, 1986. This extensively illustrated history captures the excitement and trauma of the 1906 earthquake and fire.

Bob Carter. *Food Festivals of Northern California.* Helena, MT: Falcon Publishing, 1997. For the food lover traveling in America's greatest food region.

Thomas W. Chinn. *Bridging the Pacific: San Francisco Chinatown and Its People.* San Francisco: Chinese Historical Society of America, 1989. This thoroughly researched study gives you Chinatown's inside story.

Randolph Delehanty. *San Francisco: The Ultimate Guide.* San Francisco: Chronicle Books, 1995. Delehanty is the dean of San Francisco guidebook authors, and this is the most complete guide to the city by the bay.

Rasa Gustaitis and Jerry Emory. *San Francisco Bay Shoreline Guide.* Berkeley: University of California Press, 1995. A superb guide to the natural and manmade wonders of the bay shoreline.

Don Herron. *The Dashiell Hammett Tour.* San Francisco: City Lights Books, 1991. The definitive guide to novelist Hammett's—and his legendary detective Sam Spade's—San Francisco.

Rand Richards. *Historic San Francisco: A Concise History and Guide.* San Francisco: Heritage House, 1991. Includes not only a readable history of the city, but a series of fascinating tours organized around that history.

Michael Elsohn Ross. *A Kid's Golden Gate!: Guide to Family Adventures in the National Parks at the Golden Gate.* San Francisco: Golden Gate National Parks Association, 1997. Discover the natural wonders of the Bay Area with your children.

Patricia Unterman. *Patricia Unterman's Food Lover's Guide to San Francisco.* San Francisco: Chronicle Books, 1997. An essential guide to San Francisco's astonishing culinary offerings.

Bonnie Wach. *San Francisco As You Like It: 20 Tailor-Made Tours for Culture Vultures, Shopaholics, Java Junkies, Fitness Freaks, Savvy Natives, and Everyone Else.* San Francisco: Chronicle Books, 1998. A fun and eclectic guide to San Francisco's attractions.

Sally and John Woodbridge. *San Francisco Architecture.* San Francisco: Chronicle Books, 1992. A thorough and useful guide to the city's built environment.

Films

Barbary Coast (1935); *Birdman of Alcatraz* (1962); *Bullitt* (1968); *The Conversation* (1974); *Dark Passage* (1947); *Dirty Harry* (1971); *Escape from Alcatraz* (1979); *Flower Drum Song* (1961); *The Joy Luck Club* (1993); *The Lady from Shanghai* (1948); *The Maltese Falcon* (1941); *Mrs. Doubtfire* (1993); *Pacific Heights* (1990); *The Presidio* (1988); *San Francisco* (1936); *Sister Act* (1990); *Towering Inferno* (1974); *Until the End of the World* (1991); *Vertigo* (1958)

Note: For a more complete listing of movies set in San Francisco, see Dave Monks' *The San Francisco Movie Map* (San Francisco: The Reel Map Company, 1996).

Appendix F: Local Walking Clubs and Tours

Walking Clubs

Bay Bandits Volksmarch Club
59 Convent Court
San Rafael, CA 94901

The Bay Bandits Volksmarch Club is part of the American Volkssport Association, a network of clubs that sponsor non-competitive walking, swimming, and biking events.

To receive a free general information packet that explains volkssporting and the American Volkssport Association, call the AVA at 1-800-830-WALK and leave your name, address, and phone number.

The AVA office can also give you the local phone contact for the Bay Bandits Volksmarch Club. Many AVA clubs sponsor one-day, 5K and 10K (6.2 miles) walking events, and the AVA has the dates and locations of these walks.

San Francisco Walking Tours

Chinese Cultural Heritage Foundation
Offers heritage and culinary walks through Chinatown.
415-986-1822

www.c-c-c.org

City Guides
Features free tours throughout the city led by well-informed volunteers.
415-557-4266

Dashiell Hammett Tour
Discover the favorite San Francisco spots of private eye Sam Spade—and Spade's creator, Dashiell Hammett.
510-287-9540

Foundation for San Francisco's Architectural Heritage
Explore the city's architecturally significant neighborhoods.
415-441-3004
www.sfheritage.org

Golden Gate Park
Friends of Recreation and Parks lead tours through the park much of the year. Includes tours designed for disabled access.
415-221-1311
www.frp.org

Javawalk
Offers 2-hour caffeine tour of North Beach, Chinatown, and Union Square.
415-673-WALK (9255)
www.javawalk.com

San Francisco Mural Walks
Precita Eyes Mural Arts Center
Leads you past the Mission District's more than 80 murals.
415-285-2287
www.precitaeyes.org

San Francisco Strolls
Features 26 walks customized to the character of each distinctive neighborhood.
415-282-7924

Wok Wiz/Chinatown Walking Tours
Offers cultural and culinary tours of Chinatown.
415-981-8989 or 415-981-5588
www.mim.com/wokwiz

Index

Page numbers in *italics* refer to photos

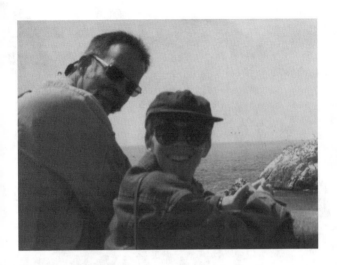

Meet the Authors

Liz Gans grew up in the San Francisco Bay Area and spent many years in San Francisco, working as marketing director for Banana Republic and The Gap. Since moving to Montana, she has directed a visual arts museum, designed databases, and worked as a management consultant. She is president of Zadig, L.L.C., and loves to walk the hills of San Francisco.

Rick Newby, until recently editorial director of Falcon Publishing, is a poet, essayist, and editor. His previous guidebooks include *Great Escapes: Montana State Parks* (Falcon, 1989), and he edited—with Suzanne Hunger—the collection of essays, *Writing Montana: Literature under the Big Sky* (1996). A relatively recent convert to the pleasures of walking San Francisco, Newby is a veteran walker. His most recent book of poems is entitled *Old Friends Walking in the Mountains.*

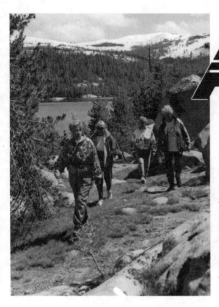

A WHOLE DIFFERENT KIND OF

Experienc
A Whole
Different
Kind of
Walk

*The American Volkssport Association,
America's premier walking organization,
provides noncompetitive sporting events for
outdoor enthusiasts. More than 500 volkssport
(translated "sport of the people") clubs sponsor
walks in scenic and historic areas nationwide.
Earn special awards for your participation.*

**For a free general information packet,
including a listing of clubs in your state,
call 1-800-830-WALK (1-800-830-9255).**

 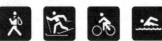

*American Volkssport Association is a nonprofit, tax-exempt,
national organization dedicated to promoting the benefits of
health and physical fitness for people of all ages.*